Chautauqua Springs, Kansas

This book is made up with several writings

from different people beginning in 1881.

It also has several pictures taken

Over the years for one to enjoy

July 2017

E STAR　　　　　　　　　　　　　　　　　　Oct. 1, 2008

Sheriff's Department finds handgun after Lackner manhunt

After intensive search, the Chautauqua County Sheriff's Department recovered a stolen 357 Magnum on Sept. 17. It was found almost one month after the capture of Robert Lackner and Erin D. Fraser, both of Kansas City, Kan., on Aug. 19 following a manhunt near Sedan.

Sheriff Frank Green and his team spent several days scouring over 800 acres of pasture, brush and dense woodlands searching for the weapon where the couple was nabbed. The weapon was fully loaded with six high performance rounds described as "cop killers".

Finding the weapon added a new charge to the list of charges from crimes allegedly committed in Kansas and Oklahoma. The new charge is possession of a firearm by a convicted felon.

The weapon is being transferred to Topeka to be tested at the KBI Ballistics Lab to determine if has been used in other crimes. One of the law enforcement officers likened the search to finding a needle in the haystack.

Lackner and Fraser still remain in jail awaiting trial.

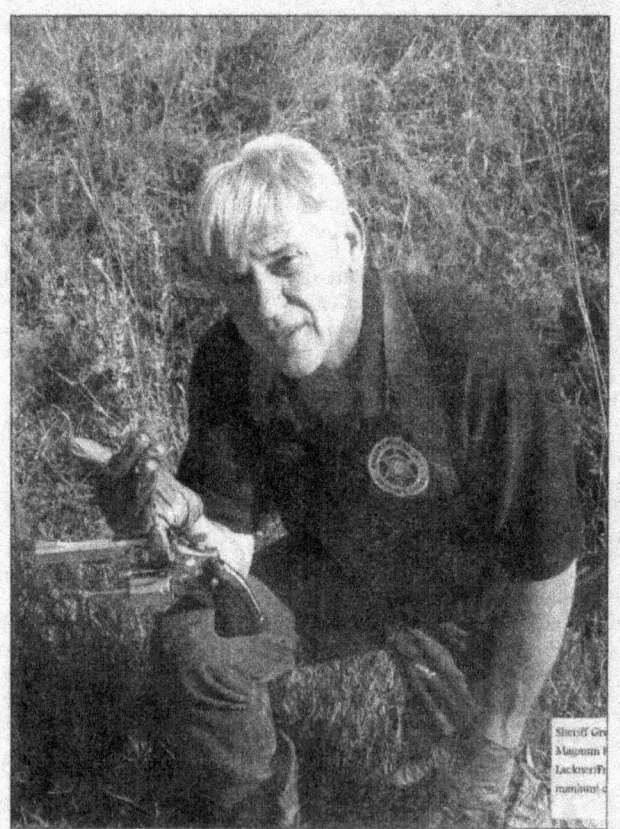

Chautauqua County Sheriff Frank Green holds the handgun used in crimes allegedly committed by Robert Lackner and Erin Fraser last month.

Kenneth & Bobbie Green Owners of Chautauqua Springs located in Chautauqua, Kansas

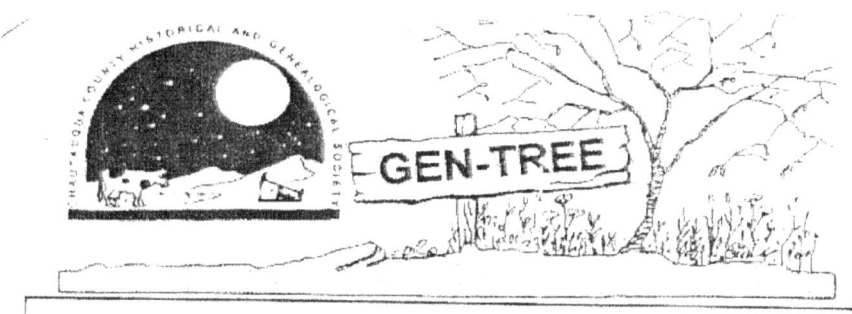

Newsletter of the Chautauqua County Historical and Genealogical Society
Web Page: http://www.imagestation.com/album/?id=4292517423
Mailing List: http://lists.rootsweb.com/index/other/Genealogical_Societies/KSCCHGS.html

| Volume 10 | January 2009 | Number 31 |

SPRINGS WERE BIG ASSET TO CHAUTAUQUA IN EARLIER DAY

(Note: The following history of Chautauqua is reproduced from a booklet advertising the town published in 1905.)

Chautauqua Springs is a thriving little village of 600 inhabitants situated in the southern part of Chautauqua County, being only one and one half miles from the line dividing Kansas and the Osage reservation.

In 1881 some of the pioneers conceived the idea that a trading point established at some place in that vicinity, which at even that early date was famed for its fertile valleys and rich pasture lands, would be a profitable investment, and eventually emerge into a thriving business center.

Their hopes have been realized and today Chautauqua is one of the best trading points and shipping stations for stock of all kinds, on the Osage line.

For years, during the shipping season, cattlemen from the immense pastures of the Osage reservation, found it advantageous to drive the stock to Chautauqua and ship. For months cattle are shipped from here by the train loads.

One of the main points of benefit of this town is the quality of water to be found in the numberless springs, from which the town derives its name. Ever since the Osage Indians were removed from Kansas to the present reservation, the healing power of this water has been known all over the central part of the United States.

Great bands of Indians, in the early days, bringing some noted chief or warrior to these springs to be healed were very common occurrences. The springs have been cleaned out, renovated, furnished so that today, despite the great influx of people owing to the great oil fields being developed, it is the best advertisement through the central states that the city has.

Following is the chemical analysis of the Chautauqua Springs mineral water made by the state chemist in 1883: Calcium sulphate 4,047; Calcium bicarbonate

3,849; magnesium 2,986; sodium 1,015; iron 1,455; sodium chloride 3,295; potassium sulphate 1,181; silica 1,633; magnesia bicarbonate trace; organic, volatile material 163. All quantities are in grains per gallon.

STATE OF KANSAS
GENERAL BALLOT
SECOND DIVISION
DISTRICT, COUNTY AND TOWNSHIP TICKET
List of Candidates to be Voted for in the County of Chautauqua.
November 7, 1950

To vote for a person, mark a cross x in the square at the right of the party name or political designation	To vote for a person, mark a cross x in the square at the right of the party name or political designation
Representative, 49th District, (Vote for one)	**Supt. Of Public Instruction,** (Vote for one)
Merle L. Lemert, Sedan, ...Republican ☐	Catharine Sturges, Sedan, ...Republican ☐
.... ☐	.... ☐
County Clerk, (Vote for one)	**Clerk of Dist. Court,** (Vote for one)
Lee Call, Sedan..................Republican ☐	Edith K. Ross, Sedan, ...Democrat ☐
.... ☐	.... ☐
County Treasurer, (Vote for one)	**County Commissioner, 1st Dist.,** (Vote for one)
M. L. Jones, Sedan..............Republican ☐	C. B. Cable, Cedar Vale, ...Rep ☐
Roy Anderson, Wauneta, ...Democrat ☐	.... ☐
.... ☐	**TOWNSHIP TICKET**
Register of Deeds, (Vote for one)	Trustee (Vote for one)
Ruby M. Polk, Sedan,..........Republican ☐	Russel Graves, Wauneta,............Rep. ☐
.... ☐	.... ☐
County Attorney, (Vote for one)	Treasurer (Vote for one)
Gerald Cauldwell, Sedan,......Republican ☐	.... ☐
.... ☐	Clerk (Vote for one)
Probate Judge, (Vote for one)	.... ☐
Ima L. Raybourn, Sedan, ...Republican ☐	**Justice of Peace** (Vote for two)
.... ☐	Ray Foster, Cedar Vale, ... ☐

May 19, 1882

Taken From the Topeka Daily

Chautauqua Quirks: Chautauqua Springs, May 12, 1882: I am preparing myself to "Preach the Gospel according to Saint John", and though I am a Greenbacker, politically, I can't help thinking the issue will be prohibition and anti prohibition this fall, and while I don't expect to abandon the principalities of the G. B. party, at least till something better is presented, I will say that I would rather be a voter for John P. John, and an advocate of the principles that he enunciates, than to see the national debt paid by a revenue obtained by and through the sale of that stuff that makes demons out of men..

I know of a good many prohibition Greenbackers that will vote for Saint John if he is nominated, and will lift every pound they can place him where he belongs. But if Saint John is not the candidate it is my opinion that the anti's-prohibition, and vise versa. If they oppose St. John they are anti-prohibitionists, at least, if they talk it is only from the teeth out.

Don't forget to send what facts and figures you can, and oblige.

Yours Respectfully, J. W. Alexander

Chautauqua Springs, Kansas

March 27, 1885

Independence, Kansas paper re: Chautauqua Springs, Kansas 1800's

Our neighboring and picturesque little city of Chautauqua Springs has recently been shaken from center to circumference by scandal of no mean dimensions, in which a handsome young lady residing in the suburbs (whose name it is not necessary to give) And Steve Johnson are the sole actors. It seems that the lady in the case was taking baths at the spring bath house for some real or imaginary disease and that Mr. Johnson had this building in his charge and that during her frequent visits to this institution, a sort of social intercourse grew up between them increasing at each subsequent visit and finally developing into a case of illicit love and the visits to the bath house became more frequent and prolonged. It is claimed by Johnson that the subjects of conversation during these visits were temperance and religion. But his wife recently found a letter in his coat pocket from the young lady confessing her undying love for him, and also one in answer to it, which Mr. Johnson had not mailed, stating that as soon as he could get a divorce from his wife he would marry the young lady and that then they would know the real meaning of true happiness. His wife thinks that religion and temperance were a kind of second consideration. At all events she turned loose with all terror and determination of a wronged and neglected wife since which time the bath house visits have been discontinued and the participants seem to have lost all interest in the cause of temperance and religion.

Mr. Johnson is one of the owners of Chautauqua Springs town site, and has always been considered one of the most moral and chaste men in the county. He is known as a rabid prohibitionist and at one time organized a law and order society at the Springs for the purpose of ridding the town of immoral and improper characters. He came forward at a revival meeting held at the Springs a few weeks ago and professed to have found Jesus. But subsequent developments go to show that it was a case of mistaken identity, it was the devil he had caught on to. To make our story end in a becoming manner, we will add that Mr. Johnson's own law and order society have given him twenty days in which to shape up his business and leave town, and we hope they will insist on having the order obeyed. He has proven himself unworthy of their society, and should be compelled to leave the community whose decency he has grossly insulted.

The Daily Commonwealth of Topeka, Kansas Sept. 17, 1886.

The Ladies Excursion

The U., V., I., and W. road was turned over to the Missouri Pacific recently and is now being operated to Leroy. Union the occasion of the first train going through, an excursion party of Independence gentlemen made the trip. The ladies being left at home were highly incensed. A fair correspondent of The Commonwealth furnishes the following incidents of the trip.

To assert our entire independence, the ladies, through the kindness of Mr. Hynes and Mr. Robinson, had a special car ran to Chautauqua Springs, thirty five miles away. The excursion was a perfect success every way and the ladies feel about two points ahead. The people of Chautauqua Springs received us with the greatest kindness, placing their hacks (all they had) at our disposal. About twenty of the ladies went across the border into the Osage nation. For real fun that was a trip which took the cake and the frosting which dripped off the edge of the baking pan. We came home at seven o'clock p.m. with our hands full of ferns, mosses and flowers.

Our correspondent adds that the ladies sent a dispatch back to their husbands and the naughty newspaperman put in more than they sent.

The enclosed clipping from a newspaper contains the following paragraph to which allusion is probably made:

The wives of Chautauqua are very busy just now driving their husbands into the brush but promise the ladies a cordial reception as soon as their worl is disposed of. A guard is about to be placed over the telephone office, and a committee has been appointed to spot reporters.

Independence, Kansas Daily Reporter September 20, 1886.

Clate Ralstin and family visited Chautauqua Springs on Friday. Clate pronounces the whole thing a failure—says there were only about one hundred fifty people present and that he could carry on his back all the contents of the agricultural hall. We rather suspect that Clate went down as a competitor for the handsomest baby premium and failed to get it, hence these unkind remarks.

Sedan Graphic: Oct. 1, 1886

About sixty five ladies of Independence took an Excursion to Chautauqua Springs. It is said that that the women at the Springs ran their husbands to the "brush" when the excursionists landed.

June 7, 1887

The excursion to Chautauqua Springs got off in fine shape this morning—or part of it. About one hundred would be excursionists were left behind owing to the fact that the train pulled out ten or fifteen minutes ahead of time and while three busses loaded down with people were just nearing the depot.

We presume that the train left ahead of time because the six passenger coaches Were already packed full of people and there were no other cars available. It is unfortunate that more cars were not provided but probably no one is to blame in the matter. The committee of course did not wish to pay for more cars than were needed and of course had to base their order on the number of tickets sold. The trouble is that people delay in purchasing tickets until the last minute thus putting at fault all previous calculations and it is to be regretted that some of the arrangement was not made by which those who purchased their tickets on time could have been protected and those only left behind who crowded in at the last minute.

The excursionists will undoubtedly have a pleasant trip and a good time and we are sorry that all who desired to go could not do so.

After the above was in type arrangements were made for another train which left at 1:30 this afternoon, carrying those who got left this morning. They will only have two or three hours at the Springs, but will have a chance to see the country and get reasonably tired.

June 8, 1887   Indy Daily Reporter

The excursion to Chautauqua Springs yesterday was a great success and with the exception of the mistake by which a number of people were left behind in the morning, was a very pleasant affair throughout the day being a delightful one and no mishaps of importance occurred. The tickets show that the number who went from here was 617, and from Cherryvale 104, Upon arrival at the Chautauqua depot ready to carry to the springs, a mile distant, all those who were unable to walk or who preferred to ride. No program or exercises had been arranged for, but one was gotten up on the spur of the moment, as the Chautauqua people desired to give the visit ors a fitting reception , and accordingly the crowd was called together and joined in singing "Beulah Land:" as appropriate to the occasion. Then the mayor introduced Judge Lynn who received the party with an appropriate address of welcome. Responses were made by Rev. Ferrell, Rice, and Evans and by Prof. Conway and Judge Hockett. Conway drew such an eloquent picture of the future of Chautauqua Springs, that at the close of his remarks the audience felt constrained to sing "Sweet Bye and Bye" which was done with a will.

After the speaking the crowd dispersed to enjoy themselves as best they could, in which everyone seems to have been successful. The return trip was made without ant adventures of interest except to three or four boys who managed to get left at Peru, the train arriving at the depot about 8 o'clock.

Chautauqua Springs bids to become a popular resort for excursion parties. The grounds are well shaded and romantic, and if a few thousand dollars could be spent in fitting them up they would be as attractive as any in this part of the state. We have learned the financial results, but understand the receipts will at least pay the expenses which are all that was expected.

June 17, 1887 Indy

In this report of the railroad excursion to Chautauqua Springs the Cherryvale Bulletin says that "Some jealousy was shown by the Independence folks because the Cherryvale ladies were so much better looking than others present and were especially admired by the natives and Independence beaux"

This is rather a mean way of getting even on the part of the Cherryvale dude who failed to make the mash he attempted on one of our Independence belles. The grapes were sour only because they hung out of your reach.   Monsieur Reynard

September 11, 1886

The Ladies Excursion

The ladies excursion to **Chautauqua Springs** got off this morning in great shape. Some sixty or sixty five representatives of the city's voluble sweetness showed up at the depot in proper time and were whirled away for a days sport among the chiggers and bugs of Chautauqua. The silence that has fallen upon the city would be oppressive if it were not partially offset by the meeting of the democratic county convention. The present outlook is that the ladies will have a solid day's rain, which will, we fear, interfere seriously with the pleasure of their trip.

Our reporter sends us the following special dispatches from the excursion:

Bolton, 8:50 a. ma.-Excursion a big success thus far. A painful rumor is afloat that there is a man aboard the train and a committee of investigation is looking for him.

Later---The villain has just been found under a seat and was promptly pitched out of the window.

Havana, 9:40—Just after that horrid man had been thrown from the train and order restored, a shriek was heard from the rear end of the train and a ferocious rat rushed through the car. All the elevated seats were quickly appropriated, and the wildest excitement and alarm prevailed until Conductor George opened the car door and the rat jumped from the train. It is believed some malicious individual put the horrid thing on board purposely and every effort will be made to ferret out the offender.

Niota 10:05—The tunnel was passed in safety and without any of the usual incidents. It wasn't a bit interesting. The sun is shining, but a black cloud in the southwest threatens. A cyclone and most of the party wish the train had stopped in the tunnel

Peru, 10:30--- The cyclone has disappeared and everybody is happy. The few lunch baskets in the party are being rapidly emptied. Those who are not busy eating are singing :" We won't go home till morning,": but the leading musicians are eating and singing is not as good as it ought to be.

Chautauqua Springs, 11 a.m. Arrived safe and nearly on time. The natives here are utterly overcome with astonishment. The wives of Chautauqua are very busy just now driving their husbands into the brush, but promise the ladies a cordial reception as soon as their work is disposed of.

A guard is about to be placed over the telegraph office, and a committee has been appointed to spot reporters. Full particulars when we get back..

Sept. 18, 1886 Coffeyville Weekly Journal

A large number of Independence ladies had a regular "hen" excursion to Chautauqua Springs one day last week. They would not allow a male biped to accompany them. The married women in the neighborhood of the Springs heard of their coming and as a precautionary measure they corralled their husbands, drove them into the brush and held them there until the attractions from Independence had taken their departure.

Indy Daily   June 7, 1887

The excursion to Chautauqua Springs got off in fine shape this morning---or rather a part of it. About one hundred would be excursionists were left behind owing to the fact that the train pulled out ten or fifteen minutes ahead of time and while three busses loaded down with people were just nearing the depot. We presume that the train lrft ahead of time because the six passenger coaches were already packed full of people and there were no other cars available. It is unfortunate that more cars were not provided but probably no one is to blame in the matter. The committee of course did not wish to pay for more cars than were needed and of course had to base their order on the number of tickets sold. The trouble is that people delay in purchasing tickets until the last minute thus putting at fault all previous calculations and it is to be regretted that some arrangements was not made by which those who purchased their tickets in time could have been protected and those only left behind who crowded in at the last minute

The excursionists will undoubtedly have a pleasant trip and a good time, and we are sorry that all who desired to go could not do so.

After the above was in type arrangements were made for another train which left at 1:30 this afternoon carrying those who got left this morning. They will only have two or three hours at the springs, but will have a chance to see the country and get reasonably tired.

June 8, 1887, Indy Daily

The Excursion

The excursion to Chautauqua Springs yesterday was a great success and with the exception of the mistake by which a number of people were left behind in the morning was a very pleasant affair throughout, the day being a delightful one and no mishaps of importance occurred. The tickets show that the number who went from here was 617, and from Cherryvale 104. Upon arrival at the Chautauqua depot, conveyances were found in waiting ready to carry to the springs, a mile distance all those who were unable to walk or who preferred to ride. No program of exercises had been arranged for, but one was gotten up on the spur of the moment, as Chautauqua people desired to give the visitors a fitting reception and accordingly the crowd was called together and joined in singing "Beulah Land" as appropriate to the occasion. Then the mayor introduced Judge Lynn who received the party with an appropriate address of welcome. Responses were made by Reverends Ferrell, Rice, and Evans, and by Professor Conway and Judge Hockett. Conway drew such an eloquent picture of the future of Chautauqua Springs that at the close of his remarks the audience felt constrained to sing "Sweet bye and bye" which was done well. After the crowd dispersed to enjoy themselves as best they could, in which everyone seems to have been successful. The return trip was made without any adventures of interest except to three or four boys who managed to get left at Peru, the train arriving at the depot about eight o'clock.

Chautauqua Springs bids fair to become a popular resort for excursion parties. The grounds are well shaded and romantic and if a few thousand dollars could be sent in fitting them up they would be as attractive as any in this part of the state. We have not learned the financial results but understand the receipts will at least pay the expenses which is all that was expected.

Oct. 17, 1887 Indy Reporter   A Hunting Party

A party of thirteen came in from Kansas City yesterday morning enrout to the territory for a week's hunting. Among the party were Mr. T.. B. Bullene and two sons of the late W. S. Gregory. The party left yesterday morning in a special car for Chautauqua Springs where they will take teams. They were accompanied by W. M. Wade who will act as guide and interpreter..

Indy July 27, 1888   Remember

The railroad excursion and Sunday School picnic to Chautauqua Springs on Friday August 3d. Tickets 75 cents, children 50 cents. Make your preparations to go out to that lively and romantic city that day and drink the healing waters of those wonderful springs.

Chautauqua Springs

A Thriving Village that Bids Fair to Become the Metropolis of Chautauqua County---
Her Mineral Springs---The only Fair in the County this Year to be Held Here

Editor Stat and Kansan---While at Chautauqua Springs a few days ago we had the pleasure through the courtesy of her enterprising business men to take a thorough look over this "Saratoga of the West." Which we hear so much about . It's location is Picturesque and beautiful, in the southeastern portion of Chautauqua county and is perhaps the only section of the county that affords a sufficient amount of tillable land to ensure to mercantile interests a steady and thriving trade. The radius from which she draws her trade is very much larger than any town of her size in the southwest.
The farmers from the east, west, and north drive a distance of from 10 to 15 miles to the springs in order to buy the most goods for their money to which the merchants of this city

are alive and make it a special ! Point in their business to look after. From the south (Osage nation) their territory is unlimited and the special inducements which are Offered in general merchandise by the various dealers brings up the full bloods from a distance of thirty or forty miles.

Prominent among her business men are John C. Romick, proprietor of the Chautauqua House: C C. Purcell, land and loan agent: Lew Lynn, Attorney at Law, F. H. Hawkins, pension claim agent, Sipple and Pershall, dealers in general merchandise and a full line of drugs, McGuire Brothers, dealers in general merchandise and hardware, F. J. Johnson, furniture and undertaking, B. F. Barrett drugs and medicines, boots and shoes, A. C. Cadwell, general merchandise, J. E. Baker, groceries and hotel, George S. Vaughn, groceries and lunch, Jacob Kaufman, ice cream, confectionary, tobacco and cigars, McGuire Bros. and Higginbotham, livery stable, W. C. Harshbarger, meat market, Drs. T. J. Dunn and Co. druggist, George Edwards, groceries and last but not least The Chautauqua Express by Wm. Wright.

These men have made Chautauqua Springs what she is and as a matter of fact only the shrewdest business maneuvering can bring about such results as have gained for her the reputation of being the leading commercial town in the country while her older sisters have pined and are dwindling to mere nothings. As we stated before, it takes pluck and energy to accomplish these ends and when a new project is proposed that looks to the Interest of the Springs every man puts his shoulder to the wheel and it goes. One of the most important improvements now going on is the macadamizing of her principal streets. For this purpose her citizens have voted bonds to the amount of $1, 500.00 which judiciously expended will make the principal through fares of the Springs what not many towns in the state of Kansas can boast of.

The latest and perhaps the most important matter ever looking towards the Springs interest is the proposition made the people by an eastern syndicate to erect, furnish and operate one of the most modern hotels of the west, hotels at older watering places not excepted. This building, as proposed is to cost $100,000.00 and the syndicate comprises ten gentlemen from an Eastern city who propose to invest in it $10,000.00.

These however are not the only improvements that are at this time on foot. Several new churches are now building and that the hotel of which we speak will be built in the near future is an absolute certainty. Why not? Take the analysis of the waters from these Springs as made by the chemist of the State University at Lawrence and we have precisely the same elements that are contained in all the famous healing waters of the Springs more thoroughly advertised and therefore more extensively patronized. If the waters of these Springs contain the healing properties of Eureka and other Springs which are assured they do it will be a matter of only a very short time when the hotel will become a paying institution, a good investment and a great summer resort.

This being true other large investments will follow such as the erection of blocks of fine business houses suitable in which to transact the mercantile business of the Springs.

We have no hesitancy in predicting for Chautauqua Springs a marvelous growth and widespread reputation for her healing waters in the near future.

Again it becomes necessary to speak of enterprise of these people and this time in a way above all others most praiseworthy. We refer to the Chautauqua county Fair which will be held at Chautauqua Springs, Kansas on September 11, 12, 13, and 14, 1888. For five consecutive years this city has held these fairs, paying each year dollar for dollar on the premiums offered by the Association. This reminds us where is the county seat? Poor old Sedan, what with 25 cents on the dollar for her premiums offered and her fair grounds sold at a Sheriff's sale? Hence the only fair of Chautauqua county this year will be held at the Springs.

Permit the statement to be made here that perhaps not many of your readers have availed themselves of opportunities heretofore presented to take a trip to this picturesque little city. To these we would say that on August 3 there will be a grand excursion fom Independence to the Springs and return for only 75 cents the round trip, half fare tickets 50 cents which may be the only excursion of the season. If you would spend the day pleasantly among hospitable people, cooling shades and medicinal sparkling waters by all means take in this excursion. Dew.

Indy Weekly Star Feb. 28, 1890

Mrs. A. C. Cadwell of Chautauqua Springs went to the Osage Agency on Tues. and had his examination before the U. S. Commissioner. Cadwell had been arrested charged with selling whiskey in the Indian Territory. The complaining witness when called at the examination testified that at the time he swore to the complaint he was so drunk that he did not know what he was doing and that some of Cadwell's enemies at Chautauqua Springs had induced him to swear to the lying complaint. Of course Mr. Cadwell was released at once. There must be some rather queer people in and about Chautauqua Springs. Sedan Times Journal.

Weekly Star, Indy June 6, 1890

For a small the following from the Cedar Vale Star, if true shows a pretty good record for bad conduct: Only six state cases this coming term of court and Chautauqua Springs furnishes all of them. Three of them for violation of the prohibitory law, two for running gambling houses and one for borrowing a horse and forgetting to return it.

From Baxter Springs, Kansas Sat. October 11, 1890

The Largest Deer on Record
The following letter from Dr. J. M. Duncan fully explains itself:

Chautauqua Springs, Kansas October 4, 1890

C. D. Meserve, Esq., Captain of Baxter Springs Gun Club, Baxter Springs, Kansas.

Dear Sir: I have just returned from two days visit among the rocky cliffs and deep canyons of the Happy Hunting Grounds of America in company with four others. The results are, three fine deer, two large turkey gobblers, plenty of fish and other small game. One of the party is suppose to have slain the largest deer on record. His gross weight was 325 pounds. From the tip of the nose to the point of hooves of the hinder feet measured eleven feet and eight inches. The antlers were in circumference at the base five and one half inches. Each antler measured thirty four and one half inches from base to tip of main shaft and each carried seven spikes, two of which on each antler measured ten inches in length each. The cut of clear tallow all over the ribs was a full half inch thick and on the saddle of the croup was one and three forth inches deep.

This animal was weighed and dressed by Mr. John Harshbarger, a butcher of Chautauqua, Springs, Kansas and the measuring was done at the camp near where he was slain and while the body was yet warm and supple by Yours truly, J. M. Duncan

Weekly Star Indy March 9, 1894

Mr. Fritch informs us that while over in Chautauqua county on Tues, he saw where a dwelling about three miles this side of Chautauqua Springs had been wrecked by Sunday night's cyclone. It was the home of a man by the name of Harris.

Indy Reporter August 29, 1896

Dr. Wright writes us the people of Chautauqua Springs invite Junior Endeavors to a beef roast at the Springs next week on Thursday. The doctor is trying to get one fare for the round trip. A big hotel will be free for sleeping. Full notice in Sunday's Reporter. Look for it.

Independence Daily Reporter May 29, 1905

Parties who wish to have Chautauqua Springs Mineral Water:
Will have to send their direct to the factory.
We will guarantee that you get the best and most prompt services and will send you nice fresh water.
Your business Earnestly Solicited.

Chautauqua Springs M. W. Co.

Indy August 1, 1905 Indy

Why Drink Impure Water. when you can get the celebrated Chautauqua Springs Mineral Water delivered at your door at a nominal cost. The medical properties of these springs were first discovered by the Big Hill and Osage Indians over forty years ago who made frequent trips to the springs for the treatment of their sick and diseased . Since that time the eater has grown famous until at the present time the water is bottled and shipped to many different parts of the United States.

The following is a description of the mineral water of Chautauqua Springs and a list of a few of the many diseases which it is adapted to the treatment of.

Temperature of the water is 58degrees Fhr, and flow is 180 gallons per hour.

The medicinal properties of this water are peculiarly adapted to this cure of rheumatism, neuralgia, nervous affections, malarial , liver and kidney diseases, sore eyes and and all kinds of skin diseases.

This mineral water is a specific cure for all chronic diseases, lung disorders, catarral affections, and fever sores of long standing, cancer, white swelling, and is unequalled for stomach troubles, etc.

Your wants will be quickly supplied by leaving your order with Scott Brothers. Local agents. Phone 118, Independence, Kansas, Kansas. 105 Penn Ave.

Independence Daily Reporter Aug. 29, 1908

Spent Night With Starr

Of all his experiences during the ride to escape the pursuing horsemen the one which seems to have impressed Coleman the most was the night he says he spent with Henry Starr in a deserted farm house in the Osage hills. He tells how at dusk, Tenant and he rode up to a barn to spend the night, they found three horses standing in the stable, saddle and bridled, Cautiously the two men climbed up in the hay loft and there sleeping on the hay was Starr, Wilson and the third member of the gang. Coleman said he could have killed all three of them as they lay there asleep. The five bank robbers spent the night together, separating at early dawn the following day.

Independence Daily Reporter Aug. 29, 1908

Clue caused Arrest

The answer came back that Coleman had been there but had left and nothing more was learned of the suspected bandits whereabouts until a message came from Washington sheriff saying that he had arrested him. Coleman .had made his first stay at Colton very short. He crossed the British Columbia and roamed around for the next month or two. The first of August he returned to his first stopping place in Washington. He was working in the wheat fields when arrested by the sheriff of Whitman county.

Why Coleman ever gave Tenant his name and destination is not known and no cause can be assigned to this act except for friendship sake. Coleman never expected to see his former pal again and no intimation was made by either that they would carry out a second bank raid together. The 'Let me hear from you' instinct is thought to have been the only purpose which led Coleman to divulge his destination to his recently acquired friend and bandit, Bill Tenant.

Coleman says he was in Chautauqua Springs only twice before the bank raid was pulled off. The first time was about ten days before the robbery to buy two horses and saddles foe him and Tenant. Coleman it seems financed the raid and paid all expenses of equipping both men. The second visit was made the morning of the day prior to the holdup when he went into the town to get the lay of the land. Coleman says that he came to Chautauqua county from Nebraska where he had previously been employed as a farm hand and that he did not know a person in Chautauqua county before coming there. He had lived in that county only five months when the raid was made.

Just A Slip of Paper

Coleman's name and address found in hid pal's pocket.

Aftermath of the Chautauqua Bank Robbery—Coleman spent one night with Henry Starr-Gave Bill Tenant his name and address.

The one big mistake of my life says Harry Coleman, the self confessed robber of the Chautauqua Springs bank in jail in the Chautauqua county jail at Sedan, was committed when I gave Bill Tenant my name and address when we parted company last spring at Kansas City. I believe had it not been for this blunder I would still have my freedom.

When Bill Tenant, the second member of the party of two who held up the bank last spring, was captured in May at Denver, a paper was found on an inside pocket with the name and destination of Harry Coleman written on it. At first Tenant would not tell who Coleman was and why he had taken his name and address, but finally Sheriff Ricketts secured a confession. The sheriff at Cotton, Whitman county Washington, was immediately wired to capture and hold Coleman.

Sept. 6, 1908

Two Boy Bandits Who Robbed Chautauqua Bank Sentenced to 10 to 20 Years in Reformatory   Sedan, Kansas. Sept. 5, 1908

Bill Tennent and Harry Coleman, the young bandits who robbed the Chautauqua State Bank at Chautauqua Springs this county on the morning of April 17 last and locked Cashier Waterhouse and Del Easley, a customer, in the vault, entered a plea of guilty in Judge Aikman sentenced each of them to from five to twenty one years in the state reformatory at Hutchinson. On account of their extreme youth and the fact that they are both very   penitent, Country Attorney Meriz asked that they be sent to the reform school instead of the penitentiary. The boys rode into Chautauqua Springs early on the morning of April 17, hitched their horses in the rear of the bank building and stepped into the bank. They immediately covered Cashier Waterhouse and Mr. Easley with large revolvers, produced a large sack and ordered the cash on hand to be placed therein. The cashier turned something over $3, 000.00 over to them. After getting what money there was in the vault they locked the cashier and Easily in the vault and walked out. Just before they concluded their job a young lady passed the door , saw what was taking place and immediately gave the alarm. The robbers in the meantime had left the bank, mounted their horses and started for the high hills south of there. Sheriff Ricketts was at once notified and with a posse started in pursuit . On account of high water at the time they soon gave up the chase but never ceased working in an endeavor to get them located.

Tennent was first captured in Denver, Colo. And on August 9, Coleman was arrested in the state of Washington. Upon the advice of Sheriff Ricketts, who had learned of his whereabouts through the aid of the postal authorities. Tennent showed no emotion whatsoever when he was sentenced this morning, but Coleman was much affected. . .

Brutes Were Bound Over   Sept. 30, 1910

Men who maimed a Chautauqua Springs Hotel keeper must answer to court.

Some time ago this paper printed a story from Chautauqua Springs telling of a brutal attack upon E. W. Jerrels hotel keeper there by three men who demanded whiskey and started in to cut Jerrels to pieces because he would not provide it. They not only beat him up badly and cut him in various places but one of them gouged out one of Jerrels eyes. The Sedan Times Star gives the story of the preliminary hearing: Elmer Higgins, Charles Hessert and Marrett Clawson were all bound over to the district court Wednesday for trial on a charge of maiming and assaulting C. W. Jerrels at Chautauqua two weeks ago. Each of them gave in bond the sum of $1,000.00.

The state alone presented evidence at the hearing at Chautauqua Wednesday before W. W. Byers, a justice of the peace. Higgins and Hessert were represented by W. H. Sproul and Clawson by D. McBrian. After the state had provided the material charge the defendants decided to offer no evidence and gave bond for their appearance at the December term of court. A large crowd attended the hearing. The state was presented by J. W. Mertz, county attorney.

The Bank Fails   Jan 27, 1915

A BANK FAILS TO OPEN DOORS

THE CASHIER OF CHAUTAUQUS SPRINGS HAS ABSCONDED
FORGERIES AMOUNT TO 420,000.00

S.E. TURNER, THE CASHIER, LEFT MONDAY MORNING SAYING HE WAS GOING TO CANEY AND HAS NOT BEEN HEARD FROM

The Citizen's State Bank of Chautauqua Springs, a little town in Chautauqua county, 40 miles due west of Coffeyville, failed to open it's doors this morning. The cashier of the situation, s. e. turner, is missing. No official statement was given out today but it is rumored that forgeries have been discovered which amount to approximately $20,000.0 Kansas City accountants are at work on the accounts.
Mr. Turner left Chautauqua Springs Monday morning saying he was going to Caney on a litle business trip and would be back that night.

Mrs. Turner is still at Chautauqua. One of the principal stock holders in the bank is J. M. Van Deventer, grandfather of the absconding cashier.
The Chautauqua bank is about fifteen years old and has had a stormy career. Four years ago it was robbed of several thousand dollars, the bandits escaping into the Osage hills just south of that town.
Accountants were in Chautauqua today at work on the books and papers of the bank. No statement was given out by any one in authority, but it is persistently rumored that forgeries have been discovered aggregating $20,000.00. Turner has always borne a good reputation.

The Leavenworth Times   Feb. 5, 1915

LEAVES ONLY $300.00 IN BANK'S VAULT

CASHIER OF CHAUTAUQUA SPRINGS INSTUTION GOT $117,000.00 IT IS BELIEVED.

Independence, Kansas, Kan. The combined loot obtained in the dozen or more recent bank robberies in Oklahoma would aggregate but a small figure in comparison with the secured by cashier s. e. Turner, who absconded from Chautauqua Springs last week after completely wrecking the Citizens State Bank there.

According to information brought to Independence by a local resident who spent Tuesday in the vicinity of Chautauqua and who met a Kansas City victim of there ruined bank.

Cashier Turner pulled off a regular Grant Gillette affair, making a cleanup of $117,000.00 with losses distributed among depositors of the bank and at least three outside investor brokers.

The bank was capitalized at $10,000.00 and carried upwards of $40,000.00 in deposits. When the vault was searched after Turner had skipped less than $200.00 was found. Since then it has developed that one brokerage firm had advanced $35,000.00, another $25,000.00 and another $17,000.00 on worthless securities, principally forged mortgages on lands, cattle and mules.

No trace of Cashier Turner has been secured since he left Chautauqua one week ago, saying that he was going to Caney on business.

Turner's grandfather, J. M. Van Deventer, principal stock holder in the bank, declares his signature to many documents to be a forgery.

Chautauqua was once a prominent spot in the Kansas oil map and is said to be coming to the front again. It is a small village situated six miles south of Sedan and about forty miles southwest of Independence.

LIGE HIGGZZINS Caught   Dec. 13, 1915

Notorious Chautauqua County Bandit and his pal Joe Kitterman are under arrest at Pueblo, Colorado.

Lige Higgins and Joseph Kitterman alleged companions of Dr. R. C. Wades in the robbery of the Chautauqua Springs bank, have been taken into custody at Pueblo, Colorado according to a telegram received from the Colorado authorities yesterday by Sheriff Powell of Sedan. The latter officer left last night for Pueblo for the two prisoners.

When Dr. Wildes confessed to be part of a bank robbery and was sentenced to the state penitentiary for a term of from ten to twenty years. It was claimed he refused to implicate his pals. However ever since the time of his confession the authorities have been after Higgins and Kitterman. Higgins was a hunted man before the Chautauqua Springs robbery, being wanted in connection with the robbery of the Niotaze bank. Kitterman's home is at Copan, Oklahoma. Higgins being a Chautauqua county product. It is claimed that there are several other members of the gang but that none of the others had anything to do with the Chautauqua Springs job.

Lyman Ford who is said to be a member of this band of desperadoes was liberated from the county jail at Miami, Oklahoma last Wednesday by some of his pals who rode into town 'stuck up' the jail and took Ford away with them.

After the Miami delivery the Chautauqua county authorities were given a tip that an effort was to be made to rescue Dr. Wildes who was in the Sedan jail awaiting to be taken to Lancing. This trick according to the information was to be turned Thursday night of last week and on that night the jail was surrounded by a heavily armed guard. The attack on the jail was not made, however but Wilder will be watched closely until he is landed in prison.

Chief of Police received a telephone message late this afternoon from Sedan stating that Sheriff Powell who arrived in Pueblo this morning had wired back that he was unable to get the prisoners as the state of Colorado refused- to release them. They killed special Santa Fe agent in making their arrest. The two men were positively identified by Sheriff Powell as being the two men wanted for the Chautauqua Springs bank robbery.--

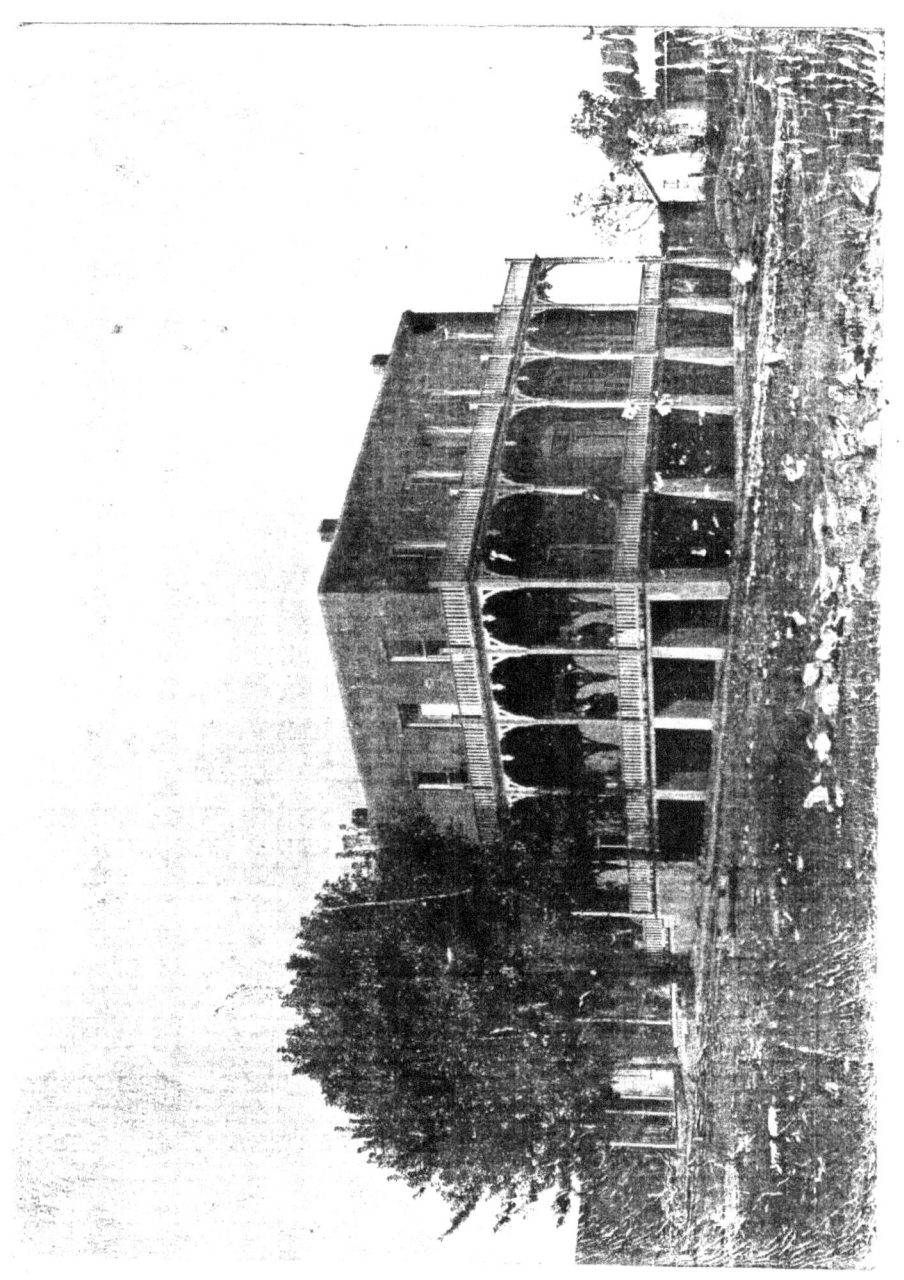

Chautauqua Springs Hotel

Spring House
Chautauqua
L side
Nora Glover
one of the owners
of Chautauqua
General Store
1897

T 48 12 H9302481.03   248   3   1
51% 172 PAGE #   PICTURE #
T 48 [c]One of the spring houses in

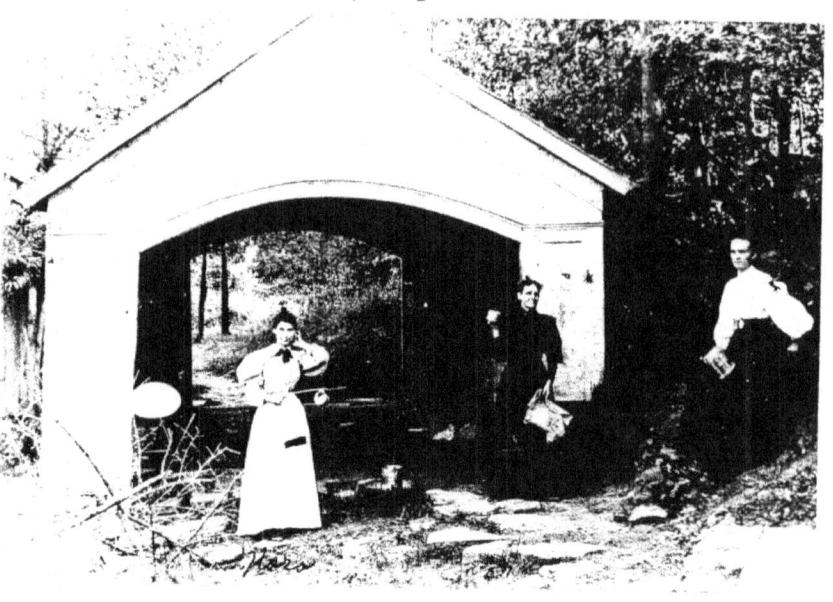

T 48 12 H9302481.03   248   2   1
56% 98 PAGE #   PICTURE #
T 48 [c]The Springs at Chautauqua so

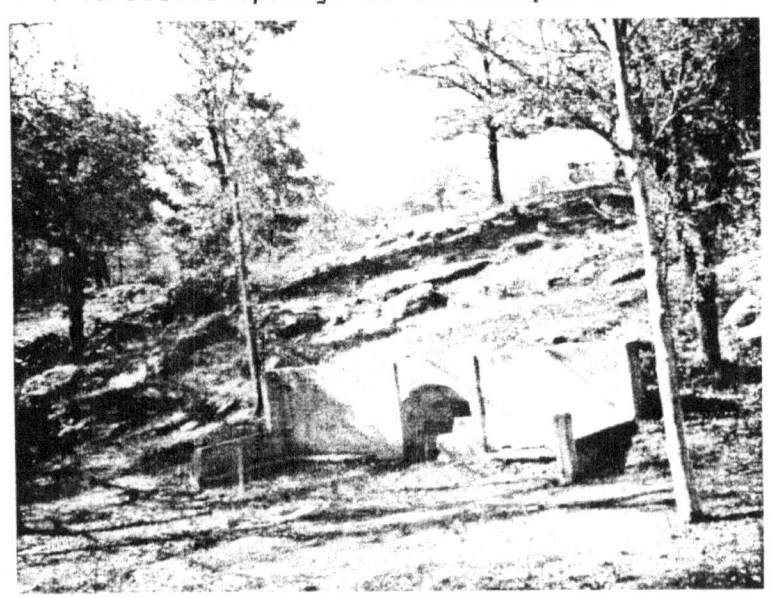

Pictures owned by Frank & Pauline Greer

THE SPRINGS

The main attraction in the city and the cause which gave rise to its building, is the presence of the mineral springs. These springs are highly valued on account of the medical properties contained in the waters, which are regarded invaluable in the cure of a variety of chronic sores and other diseases. The curative properties of these waters are known, not only through medical and chemical analysis, but are also attested by the apparently miraculous cures effected by their experimental use and application in many instances.

The discovery of these springs was made in 1873, by Dr. Minna, a physician who practiced in the vicinity at that time. It was his custom, when riding by, to drink of the water, and although recognizing the presence of mineral taste in them, yet made no further analysis. His belief during all this time, however, was that, possibly, there were in these same waters medical ingredients that might prove valuable in the healing of diseases. In the latter years of his life the Doctor was afflicted with dropsy, and for a long time was under the treatment of medical skill, from which he derived little benefit.

Finally the physicians gave up the case as incurable, and the old Doctor turning to the scriptural injunction of "Physician heal thyself," concluded, as a last hope, to try the waters which he had discovered. A quantity of the water was brought, of which he made frequent use and application, and from which he believed himself to experience much benefit. But the old man had too long been weighed down with the wasting disease, and the "treatment of physicians," to ever hope to regain health from any cause, and at length passed away, leaving, as a testimonial, his belief that had he begun the use of the water in time, he would the old man had too long been weighed down with the wasting disease, and the "treatment of physicians," to ever hope to regain health from any cause, and at length passed away, leaving, as a testimonial, his belief that had he begun the use of the water in time, he would have succeeded in removing the disease, and been restored to health.

Nothing was done toward making further test of these mineral springs until opened by Dr. G. W. Woolsey in August, 1880. The spring is neatly and substantially walled up, and is constructed with a large basin for holding the water, the whole being covered by a commodious spring house, tastefully built, paved with flag rock, and conveniently seated with benches. An analysis of the waters was made by practical chemists of some note, of the cities of St. Joseph and Kansas City, showing the water to contain, in different proportions, iron, potassium, salts and magnetic gas.

While excavating the earth, in opening up the spring, the workmen struck upon rocks, standing upright, and arranged in a sort of basin shape, presenting evidence that it had been the handiwork of man, and giving rise to the theory that perhaps one day these waters were known to some Indian tribe, who made use of them in their primitive way, for the curing of disease.

The curative properties of these springs is as yet but little known, and it is safe to predict that when their efficacy become known to the world, and a thorough test is made, hundreds will flock in to partake of the benefits of the healing fountain.

The city as yet presents an appearance of newness, the most of the houses being unpainted and scattered.

The population of the town at this time numbers about 300, to which addition is being made by the incoming of settlers almost constantly.

Analysis of Chautauqua Mineral Water Taken By State chemist of Kansas, 1882, the following is an analysis of the Mineral Water of Chautauqua Springs and a list of the many diseases which it is adapted to the treatment of:

Calcium Sulphate	4.047	grains
Calcium Bicarbonate	3,849	grains
Magnesium	2,986	grains
Sodium	1.015	grains
Iron	1.455	grains
Sodium Chloride	3.295	grains
Potassium Sulphate	1.181	grains
Silica	1.633	grains
Magnesium Bicarbonate		trace
Organic, Volatile Mat.	.163	grains
Total Constituents	19.624	grains
Cubic Gal's		

Temperature of this water is 58 degrees Fhr., and the flow is 180 gallons per hour. The medicinal properties of this water are peculiarly adapted to the cure of Rheumatism, Neuralgia, Nervous Affections, Malarial, Liver and Kidney Deseases, Sore Eyes, and all kinds of skin diseases.

This Mineral Water is a Specific Remedy for Veneral Diseases and for all Chronic Diseases, Lung Disorders,

gallons per hour. The medicinal
properties of this water are peculiarly
adapted to the cure of Rheumatism,
Neuralgia, Nervous Affections, Malarial,
Liver and Kidney Deseases, Sore Eyes,
and all kinds of skin diseases.
    This Mineral Water is a Specific
Remedy for Venereal Diseases and for

Catarrhal Affection and Feversores
of long standing, Ulcers, White Swelling
unequalled for stomach troubles, etc.

        Chautauqua Springs Mineral Water
Company
            Chautauqua, Kansas

    (Journal-Capital Print. Pawhuska)
    (Union Label)

Wonders of the World

Nature's Remedy: Queen of all Mineral Waters

Numbers of living witnesses Testify Daily to the benefits of these waters

The following diseases have no equals, Rheumatism in all it's forms, Scrofula, Skin Diseases, Kidney Troubles,
Sore eyes, Diabetes, Indigestion, Dyspepsia, Asthma, Bronchitis, Female Diseases, and Bronchitis.

When the Spring Waters were tested by State Chemists of Kansas in 1882 they analyzed the Mineral Water and stated a list of diseases which is adapted to the treatment of:

Cure of Rheumatism, Neuralgia, Nervous Affections, Malarial, Liver and Kidney Diseases, Sore Eyes, and all kinds of skin diseases.

This Mineral Water is a Specific Remedy for Venereal Diseases and for all Chronic Diseases, Lung Disorders,

Catarrhal Affection, and Fever Sores of long Standing, Ulcers, White Swelling, unequalled for stomach troubles.

Chautauqua Springs Mineral Water Company,   Chautauqua Springs, Kansas

Spring on the East side of Town Chautauqua

by Jennifer Mattocks

Beautiful hills, rocks and rolling countryside greets the visitor to Chautauqua, as he or she is coming from the east into town from the old sandhills road. That is where the springs are and the old hotel used to be.

Chautauqua once had the name "Chautauqua Springs." The springs were known far and wide for their mineral water. A large hotel was once down by the springs to accommodate the people who came for mineral baths. The spring is still there, located just east of the Southern Baptist Church.

Chautauqua has another church, The Rock Church, which was built in 1886-87 of stone from a quarry NW of town. Chautauqua was also known as the "Chapel of The Trails."

Today, in Chautauqua, there are not as many things as there used to be. There used to be a grocery store, feed store, dry goods store, general store, a grade school and high school, post office, a bank built in 1905, a city hall and the churches. Today, there is the West 80's Campground, Steve's S. 99 Stop, Christian school, the Rock Church, the Southern Baptist Church, Post Office and Senior Citizens Center.

Rumor has it that the Dalton Gang used to ride up and down Chautauqua's Main street every day. They never even attempted to rob the bank though. They would just hide in the ravines down in Oklahoma or in the old Robber's Caves in Elgin.

Chautauqua is a very quiet town to live in. At night, one can watch the sunset, a blaze of yellow, orange and red. One can sit in their back yard and watch the birds fly or just feel the cool breeze in the summer dusk.

I would suggest to anyone having time to go visit a small, quiet town, to go to Chautauqua, where the people are friendly, the scenery is beautiful and one can relax.

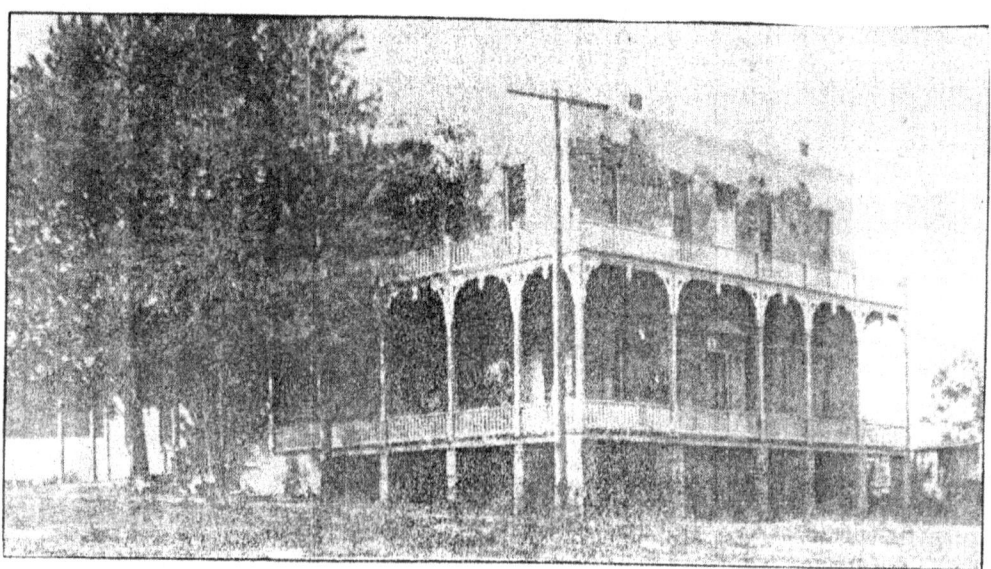

Old Chautauqua Hotel where people went to take a spring fed bath on the east side of town. Photo Credit Louise McElroy

Exclusively reaching over 4,300 homes in Chautauqua and Elk County!

Chautauqua Hotel Destroyed By Fire

Old structure caught fire about midnight Sunday and is a total loss.

~ Reprinted from The Sedan Times Star, August 4, 1929, Volume 57, No. 32 ~

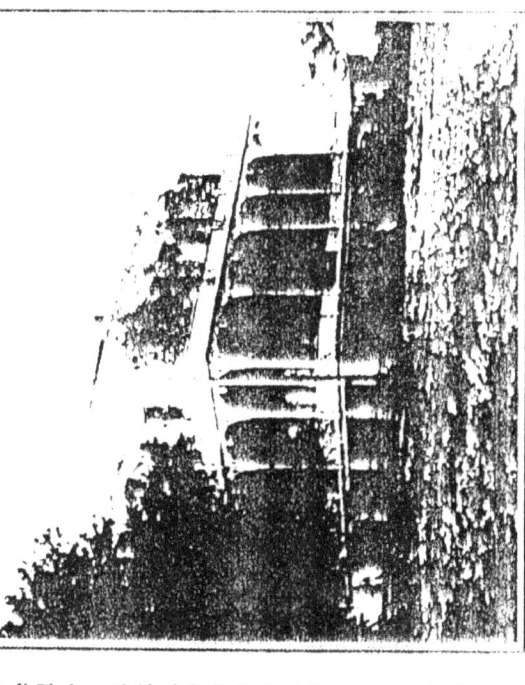

The Eagle Hotel, also known as the "Stone Hotel" was built in 1880 and was a focus of pride for the community. The hotel stood for nearly 50 years before being completely destroyed by fire in 1929.

he old stone hotel at Chautauqua Springs burned Sunday night. The building together with the nts was a total loss.

he building was unoccupied, with the exception of oom which was used by the owner, D.B. Easley, as ping room. Easley says he was awakened about ght by a noise in the building. Getting up, he d out in the yard from his window, but could see e around. His dog was barking and making a big about something, which was as much as he could ve that was out of the ordinary. Dismissing the nt, he lay down and had just relapsed into a doze he smelled smoke. Opening the door the hallway so densely filled with smoke to attempt to get out ay, so he made his exit outside through an up- window. He immediately gave the alarm, but by me assistance had arrived the fire had gained too headway to be extinguished with the apparatus ble. The cause of the blaze is a mystery; no fire g been used about the building recently for any se.

r. Easley, who is making an effort to bring auqua Springs back to popularity as a health was making plans to open up the hotel as soon ditions could justify an attempt at its operation d a quantity of furniture and furnishings stored in ilding that went up in smoke with the rest of it. d insurance on the building, which will partly his loss.

e Burning down of the old hotel building, which arge stone structure consisting of two stories and ent, marks the passing of one of the earliest landmarks in the country to achieve fame and popularity. Its fortunes had fluctuated with various booms the Springs have had since the settling of the county, and the rise and fall of many high hopes have been experienced upon its site.

The hotel was built during the early part of 1882 when Chautauqua Springs was in the heyday of its first glory. It was formally opened to the public on Sunday, June 4, 1882. Its first landlord who presided at the opening was the late Benton Smith, who moved there from Independence to operate under lease. During its late fortunes it was owned for a number of years by the late W.H. Dennis, who owned it at the time of his death. Since then it has figured in the hands of various owners as trading stock until last year it was secured by Mr. Easley to be used as a feature of his efforts to bring the Springs back to public attention and patronage.

The last person to operate it as a public hotel was Mrs. E.E. Embree of Sedan. She gave it up about six years ago, since which time it has remained idle property.

The walls of the old building were an excellent job of native stone work such as only the early day craftsmen knew how to carve, cut and lay. The interior woodwork was mostly of native lumber, oak and black walnut sawed out of the timber in that vicinity. A solid black walnut staircase of exceptionally attractive design and fine workmanship, excited the admiration of all who beheld it, and the eternal destruction of that staircase is the first comment of all familiar with it, when expressing their regret that the old landmark had gone up in flames.

From SEDAN TIMES STAR
August 4, 1929
Volume 57   No. 32

CHAUTAUQUA HOTEL DESTROYED BY FIRE
-----Old structure caught fire about midnight Sunday and is a total loss.

The old stone hotel at Chautauqua Springs burned down Sunday night. The building together with the contents was a total loss.

The building was unoccupied, with the exception of one room which was used by the owner, D.B. Easley, as a sleeping room. Easley says he was awakened about midnight by a noise in the building. Getting up, he looked out in the yard from his window, but could see no one around. His dog was barking and making a big fuss about something, which was as much as he could observe that was out of the ordinary. Dismissing the incident, he lay down and had just relapsed into a doze when he smelled smoke. Opening the door the hallway was too densely filled with smoke to attempt to get out that way, so he made his exit outside through an upstairs window. He immediately gave the alarm, but by the time assistance had arrived the fire had gained too much headway to be extinguished with the apparatus available. The cause of the blaze is a mystery, no fire having used about the building recently for any purpose.

Mr. Easley, who is making an effort to bring Chautauqua Springs back to popularity as a health resort, was making plans to open up the hotel as soon as conditions could justify an attempt at its operation. He had a quantity of furniture and furnishings stored in the building that went up in smoke with the rest of it. He had insurance on the building, which will partly cover his loss.

The burning down of the old hotel building, which was a large stone structure consisting of two stories and basement, marks the passing of one of the earliest landmarks in the county to achieve fame and popularity. Its fortunes had fluctuated with various booms the Springs have had since the settling of the county, and the rise and fall of many high hopes have been experienced upon its site.

The hotel was built during the early part of 1882 when Chautauqua Springs was in the heyday of its first glory. It was formally opened to the public on Sunday, June 4, 1882. Its first landlord who presided at the opening was the late Benton Smith, who moved there from Independence to operate under lease. During its late fortunes it was owned for a number of years by the late W.H. Dennis, who owned it at the time of his death. Since then it has figured in the hands of various owners as trading stock until last year it was secured by Mr. Easley to be used as a feature of his efforts to bring the Springs back to public attention and patronage.

The last person to operate it as a public hotel was Mrs. E.B. Embree of Sedan. She gave it up about six years ago, since which time it has remained idle property.

The walls of the old building were an excellent job of native stone work, such as only the early day craftsmen knew how to carve out and lay. The interior woodwork was mostly of native lumber, oak and black walnut, sawed out of the timber in that vicinity. A solid black walnut staircase of exceptionally attractive design and fine workmanship, excited the admiration of all who beheld it, and the eternal destruction of that staircase is the first comment of all familiar with it, when expressing their regret that the old landmark had gone up in flames.

(From historical files of Librarian and Teacher Louise McElroy-Chautauqua)

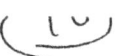

EAGLE HOTEL--CHAUTAUQUA, KANSAS
------by Louise McElroy

The Eagle Hotel in Chautauqua, Kansas, was built during the early part of 1882 when Chautauqua Springs was in the heyday of its first glory. It was a large, stone structure consisting of two stories and a basement. It was formally opened to the public on Sunday, June 4, 1882. Its first landlord who presided at the opening was Benton Smith who had moved to Chautauqua from Independence, Kansas, to operate under lease.

The Eagle Hotel was to achieve fame and popularity. Its fortunes fluctuated with various booms the Springs have had since the settling of the county. The rise and fall of many high hopes have been experienced upon its site.

During its late fortunes it was owned for a number of years by the late W.F. Dennis, who owned it at the time of his death. It then figured in the hands of various owners as trading stock until 1928 when it passed into the hands of of Mr. D.B. Easley. He used it as a feature of his efforts to bring back the Springs to public attention and patronage. After all, people had come from as far away as New York, in earlier days, to stay in the Eagle Hotel and bathe in the curative waters or drink of the health-giving water.

Prior to Mr. Easley's efforts, the last person to have operated the hotel was a Mrs. E.B. Embree of Sedan. She had given it up about 1923 after which time it had remained idle property until about 1928 to 1929. And, other than the hotel having rooms for visitors from far away, local people found it useful when they wished to stay in town for the skating activities or the musicals to be given at the Springs.

The walls of the building were an excellent job of native stone work such as only the early-day craftsmen knew how to cut and lay. The interior woodwork was mostly of native lumber, oak and walnut, sawed out of the timber in that vicinity. A solid black walnut staircase of exceptionally attractive design and fine workmanship excited the admiration of all who beheld it. When the fateful fire of August 1929 burned the hotel, the eternal destruction of that staircase brought the first words of regret among the others to be spoken concerning its burning.

Actually, during the year of 1928, Del Easley had brought about quite a revival of the Springs by hard work and effort and much publicity. For quite some time the Springs flourished. It was during this time, especially, that people from as far away as New York came to stay in the Eagle Hotel and bathe in the Springs, as well as drink the mineral water. This was short lived, however, as the Eagle Hotel burned in August of 1929, reducing it to ashes. Fire took away one of the finest hotels ever to have been in the county at that date and fire also took away the only lodging place in Chautauqua at that time.

Many older residents of Chautauqua think that A.J. Slates or his father and family helped to do the rock work of the Eagle Hotel. In 1905 Mr. A.J. Slates did rock work around the big spring and also worked on the stone school house. Stone was removed from a quarry about one-fourth mile west of Chautauqua on land then owned by the Slates family. Whether or not he did all the rock work on the hotel may be known or recorded somewhere.

From the Sedan Times Star of August 4, 1929, Volume 57, Number 32, an account appeared which bore the headline as follows:
    CHAUTAUQUA HOTEL DESTROYED BY FIRE
        ------Old structure caught fire about midnight Sunday and is a
            total loss.
(Enclosed is a copy of the news item as copied from old files.)

The Arkansas City Daily Traveler --------1928

FAME OF CHAUTAUQUA SPRINGS, NEAR SEDAN, WILL BE REVIVED

The fame once enjoyed by Chautauqua Springs, Kansas, located about ten miles south of Sedan, as the home of health-giving mineral water, is expected to be revived. Plans are on foot for the rejuvenation of the resort, the work to be done by or under the direction of Dr. D. B. Easley, owner. It is planned to make the spot a real health resort and recreation ground for Northern Oklahoma and Southern Kansas.

The Springs were at one time owned by a company headed by Dr. Easley, but the concern failed, and the prosperity of the resort ebbed. For years the Springs have lain idle, and it was only recently that Dr. Easley managed to gain sole ownership of the place. He is losing no time now to put into actual operation his new project.

In th early days when Oklahoma was still a territory, a large number of characters of early bandit history made the springs their rendevous. Henry Starr, Kid Wilson, Three Finger Jack, Bill Doolan, Cherokee Bill, the Daltons and many others drank from the springs water at one time and came back for more.

Later, about the time Oklahoma was admitted as a state, in 1907 Chautauqua Springs was known far and wide for the mineral water shipped from there. In neighboring towns, restaurant menus gave the diner choice of coffee, tea, or Chautauqua Springs mineral water. The fluid was shipped out in carload lots and hauled away in wagon loads. People by the thousands came from long distances to drink from the springs and spend their time there.

And the former fame of the place is expected to come again with the rehabilitating of the springs. The former race track, a half-mile affair, will be put in repair for use during the season. The HOTEL will be refurnished and d stuccoed and made inhabitable with modern improvements from top to bottom. Baths of all sorts with the wonderful water from the spring will be available, and the many games such as tennis, croquet, golf, and what-not, will be provided for. The zoo there will be re-established.

Teddy Roosevelt Is Guest at Chautauqua Springs Hotel

"Theodore Roosevelt, Washington, D.C." written in a bold and flowing handwriting can be seen at the Emmett Kelly Museum.

This famous visitor has registered twice in the old hotel register of the Chautauqua Springs hotel in Chautauqua, Kans.

On Sunday, March 20, 1904 and again on Aug. 20, 1904, the former president of the United States was a hotel guest.

This register boasts of many names, some more famous than others, but the names provide a key to the history of turn of century era of travel. Some became guests because of the slowness of the mode of travel in those days making it necessary for a traveler to divide his trip into many stops. Others came to seek the therapeutic promises of the mineral spa, namely, Chautauqua Springs.

Another name catching the eye is that of Booker T. Washington of Tuskogee, Ala., who signed the daily register on Feb. 6, 1906.

At this time Mrs. M. E. Edwards was manager of the Chautauqua Springs Hotel, a two-story gingerbread holstry trimmed with many white columned porches depicting the decorative art of the time.

It may be a far cry from speaking of the visit of the then president of the United States to a story of Teddy Bear, but the story of the boisterous, roughrider president is one of many facets.

In 1901 Theodore Roosevelt became the 26th president of the United States following the assassination of William McKinley. The following year he went to Mississippi to settle a minor boundary dispute between that state and the state of Louisiana.

Mr. Roosevelt drew a line between the two states. But during his stay in Mississippi, Teddy Roosevelt had gone on a hunting expedition. During the hunt he had refused to shoot a small bear cub.

This incident occurred in November of 1902, and immediately a cartoon appeared which implied that not only did Mr. Roosevelt draw the line between the two states, he also drew the line on his hunting of cub bears.

Various credits are accorded to different ones capitalizing upon this incident. One cites a Brooklyn shopkeeper and his wife who made stuffed teddy bears and put them in the shop window. They were immediately in demand.

While examining this hotel registry displayed at the local Emmett Kelly Museum, look for the signature of Theodore (Teddy) Roosevelt, and the impact of history greets the viewer as Roovevelt's flamboyant personality speaks through the pages. Each signed line and page of the register reflects a bit and piece of the history of another era reflected in today's eyes of 1972. Names from far and wide, as well as local notables appeared therein.

CHAUTAUQUA HOTEL DESTROYED BY FIRE

(Taken from The Sedan Times Star August 4, 1929)

The old stone hotel at Chautauqua Springs burned down Sunday night. The building with the contents was a total loss. The building was unoccupied, with the exception of one room which was used by the owner, D. B. Easley, as a sleeping room. Easley says he was awakened about midnight by a noise in the building. Getting up, he looked our in the yard from his window, but he could see no one around. His dog was barking and making a big fuss about something, which was as much as he could observe that was out of the ordinary. dismissing the incident, he lay down and had just relapsed into a doze when he smelled smoke. Opening the door the hallway was too densely filled with smoke to attempt to get out the way, so he made his exit outside through an upstairs window. he immediately gave the alarm, but by the time assistance arrived the fire had gained too much headway to be extinguished with apparatus available. The cause of the blaze is a mystery, no fire having been used about the building recently for any purpose.

Mr. Easley, who is making an effort to bring Chautauqua Springs back to popularity as a health resort, was making plans to open up the hotel as soon as conditions could justify an attempt at its operation. he had a quanity of furniture and furnishings stored in the building that went up in smoke with the rest of it. He had insurance on the building which will partly cover his loss. The Burning down of the old hotel which was a large stone structure consisting of two stories and basement, marks the passing of one of the earliest landmarks in the county to achieve fame and popularity. The hotel was built in during the early part of 1882 when Chautauqua Springs was in the heyday of its first glory. It was formerly opened to the public June 4, 1882. It's first landlord who presided at the opening was the late Benton Smith, who moved there for Independence to operate under lease. During its late fortunes is was owned for a number of years by the late W. H. Dennis, who owned it at the time of his death. The last person to operate it as a public hotel was Mrs. E. B. Embree of Sedan. It then was secured by Mr. Easley in 1928 to be used as a feature of his efforts to bring back the Springs back to public attention and patronage.

Wednesday, September 29, 1976   THE SEDAN TIMES-STAR

Chautauqua Main Street — This is the way Chautauqua's Main Street once looked. Harold McDowell brought us the picture post card which he believes was taken sometime during the teen years. McDowell says the picture was taken near the Walter Darnall home looking north.

33

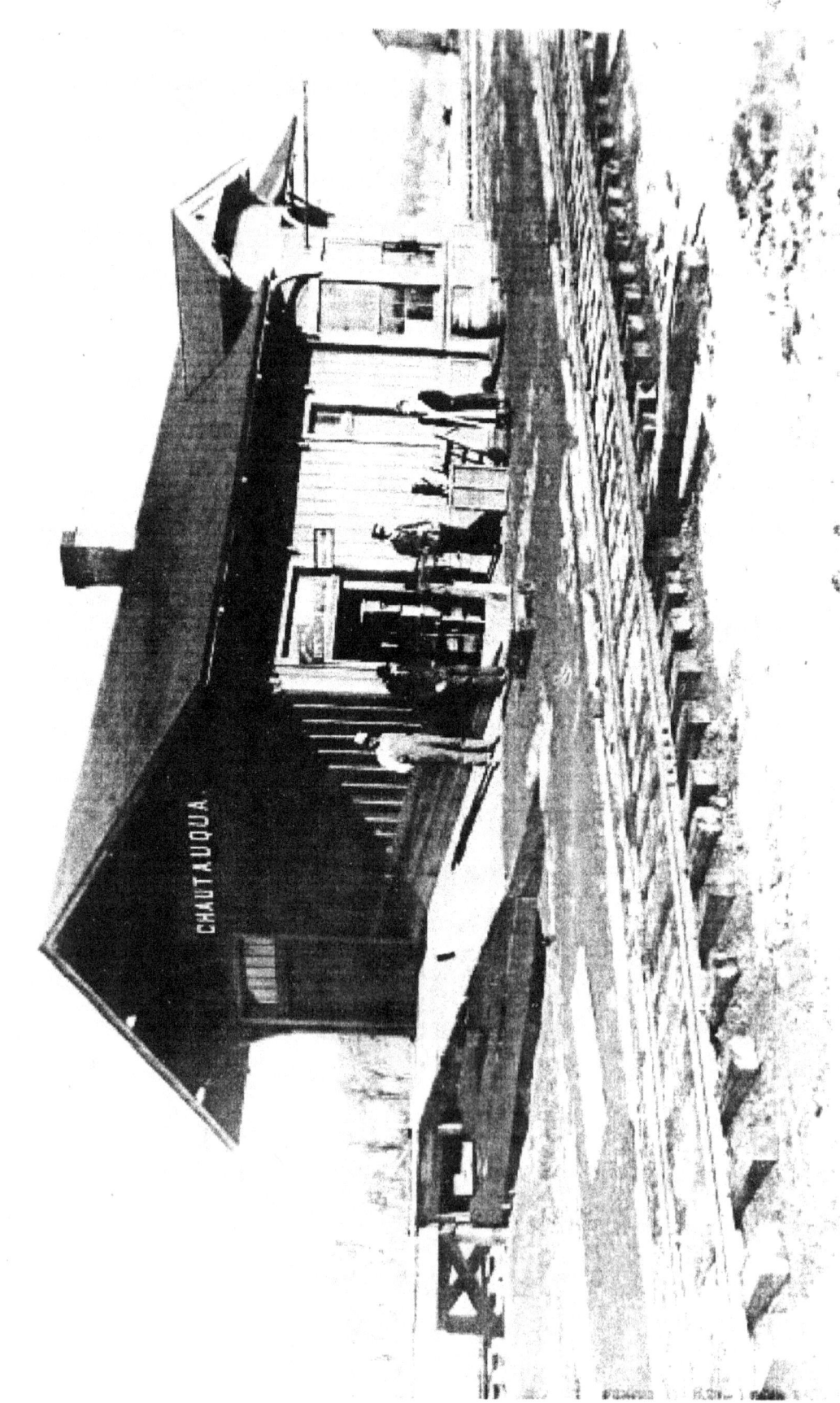

CHAUTAUQUA SPRINGS
1883
(Research notes taken from the past)

This little city sprang into existence August 10, 1881. The presence of mineral springs, highly celebrated for the medical properties of the waters, was the chief incentive to its starting.

The place is situated in the south part of Chautauqua County, about eight miles south of the city of Sedan and one mile from the picturesque Indian Territory. Its surroundings are beautiful, lying as it does on the brink of a small rocky canyon, a branch of Turkey Creek, from which stream it is a short distance. The landscape is interestingly diversified with hill, canyon, and rocky cliff, and is covered with a dense growth of shrub and timber. The city lies in the midst of a grove of forest trees, much of the timber being allowed to remain, giving it the appearance of a city in the woods.

The first house erected on the site belonged to B. F. Bennett, which he used for a drug store. Following this, during the fall, and in almost consecutive order, was the establishment of a dry goods house by T. J. Bryant, a grocery and provision story be Bennett and Binns, and a drug store by George Edwards, who was also the first postmaster in Chautauqua. In February of 1882, Dick Foster opened a store of hardware which he sold to W. Williams in September of the same year. About that time C. C. Purcell began the drug business. A grocery store belonging to James Randall was opened in October, 1881, and about the same time Mrs. Bush started a millinery establishment. James Sipples opened a drygoods store in August, 1882. Besides these, there are also two livery barns, two blacksmith shops, two wagon shops, and a sawmill belonging to James Allreid, who began the business in December, 1881.

The first hotel was built by a man named Castleberry, who ran it about six months and after changing hands several times it is still used as a hotel of which there are now three in the city. Two of these, the Ginn and Meeks houses, are small affairs; but the other, the Eagle Hotel, erected in June, 1882, by James Ferguson, is the finest public house in the county. It is a large two-story stone structure 60 feet long and 40 feet wide, containing 25 rooms for accomodations for about 60 guests. The house is constructed with long verandas on two sides, and on either floor. It stands on the slope of the canyon a few steps from the springs and overlooks the deeper canyon of Turkey Creek and the beautifully timbered hills stretching far away in the smoky distance into Indian Territory.

CHAUTAUQUA SPRINGS

1912
(Research notes taken from the past)

Chautauqua, one of the incorporated towns of Chautauqua County, is a station on the Atchison, Topeka, and Santa Fe R.R. in Bellville township, in the southern part of the county, 7 miles from Sedan, the judicial seat. It has a bank, a grist mill, a weekly newspaper (The Globe), express and telegraph offices, and a money order postoffice. It is the shipping point for a large agricultural area. The population in 1910 according to the census report was 348. The chief incentive for founding a town at this point was the mineral springs. The landscape is interesting and picturesque, and the springs are said to have great curative properties. The town was located in 1881, and by the next year there were 300 inhabitants. The first newspaper, the Chautauqua Springs Spy, was established in 1882 by C. E. Moore and L. G. B. McPherson. It had 350 subscribers. Some of the early business men who came in during the first two years were: B. F. Bennett, drugs; T. J. Johnson, drygoods; F. M. Fairbands, livery barn; Thomas Bryant, drygoods; Bennett and Binns, grocery store; George Edwards, drugs; Richard Foster, hardward; C. C. Purcell, drugs; James Randall, grocery store; Mrs. Bush, millinery; James Allreid, who owned a sawmill; Castleberry, the hotel man; and six others who established livery barns, blacksmith shops, and wagon shops. The school district was organized in 1880.

The original townsite was consisted of 80 acres, belonging to Dr. G. W. Woolsey and Dr. T. J. Dunn, to which additions were made by J. C. Kyles and Binns and Bennett. Chautauqua was incorporated as a city of the third class in 1882 and the following officers were chosen at the first election: Mayor, Thomas Bryant; clerk, S. Booth; treasurer, I. H. Wilson;

Kansas Post Offices, 1828-1961
Results of Query:

Post Office: All post offices
County: Chautauqua

Page 1 of 2 showing 50 records of 59 total, starting on record 1

Post Office	County	Established	Discontinued	Notes
Belknap	Chautauqua	1877-12-10	1878-10-29	
Belknap	Chautauqua	1872-08-28	1878-11-23	Established in Howard County.
Boston	Chautauqua	1871-08-28	1879-09-01	Moved to Moline. Established in Howard County.
Bradley	Chautauqua	1891-02-10	1894-07-31	
Brownsville	Chautauqua	1883-05-23	1903-04-30	
Cascade	Chautauqua	1882-06-26	1886-12-04	
Cedar Vale	Chautauqua	1870-05-02	Open in 1961	Established in Howard County.
Center	Chautauqua	1897-08-21	1907-02-28	
Center	Chautauqua	1871-12-01	1894-10-31	Also spelled Centre. Established in Howard County.
Chautauqua	Chautauqua	1881-10-03	Open in 1961	
Cloverdale	Chautauqua	1871-01-24	1905-04-15	Established in Howard County.
Colfax	Chautauqua	1873-12-24	1906-11-15	
Colfax	Chautauqua	1872-08-05	1873-02-24	Established in Howard County.
Elgin	Chautauqua	1887-08-12	1976-07-30	
Elgin	Chautauqua	1871-02-27	1887-07-21	Name change to New Elgin. Established in Howard County.
Farmersburg	Chautauqua	1897-12-02	1906-01-15	
Farmersburg	Chautauqua	1872-04-25	1896-02-15	Also spelled Farmerburgh. Established in Howard County.
Farmersburg	Chautauqua	1896-03-24	1896-05-15	[Order of change rescinded]
Fulda	Chautauqua	1872-08-05	1883-04-02	Name change to Wauneta. Established in Howard County.
Golden Gate	Chautauqua	1872-03-20	1876-07-03	Established in Howard County.
Grafton	Chautauqua	1888-01-18	1906-10-31	
Grafton	Chautauqua	1871-04-05	1887-10-01	Established in Howard County.
Hale	Chautauqua	1882-05-18	1907-06-29	
Hart's Mill	Chautauqua	1872-06-03	1887-04-06	Moved to Hewins. Established in Howard County.
Hewins	Chautauqua	1887-04-06	1966-04-08	Moved from Hart's Mill.
Jay Hawk	Chautauqua	1871-04-05	1871-09-01	Name change to Matanzas. Established in Howard County.
Jonesburg	Chautauqua	1892-06-08	1903-08-31	Name change from Jonesburgh.
Jonesburgh	Chautauqua	1877-11-21	1892-06-08	Name change to Jonesburg.
Leeds	Chautauqua	1883-08-06	1927-01-31	Name change from Squib.
Lisbon	Chautauqua	1872-04-29	1880-09-15	Established in Howard County.

began raising cotton. He also built a cotton gin in the vicinity. The town of Cascade no longer exist.

CEDAR VALE The origin of Cedar Vale dates back to the arrival of J. R. Marsh, 25 year old New Yorker in 1869, he determined the present location of Cedar Vale, would be ideal for a town site. Other enterprising settlers began to arrive, and the matter of establishing a town was talked of among these parties and finally a town company was organized in 1870. The name of Cedar Vale was adopted because of the Cedars growing along the creek. The first post office was established in 1870, The first stock of merchandise was brought in 1869 and was sold out to Indians. In 1870, Mr. Marsh started work on the first store building, Riley Bros, built the second store building, Luke Phelps built a box house 14X24 and used it for a hotel, and Riley Bros, built another house. These four building were the only ones in Cedar Vale at the close of 1870.

Cedar Vale grew to a thriving community with many business establishment on main street, a large school, two grain elevators, a livestock auction house, cafes, a hospital, bank and the post office is still operational. Cedar Vale has a very large, interesting museum which will take you back into its early days.

CENTRE was established in Lafayette township in 1871. During Centre's existence they boasted a grist mill, two churches, a school, a general store and hotel. The post office at Centre was closed in 1907. Today there are no signs of the town site.

CHAUTAUQUA SPRINGS OR CHAUTAUQUA was a thriving little village of 600 inhabitants situated in the southern part of Chautauqua County, living only one and one half miles from the line dividing Kansas and the Osage reservation. In 1881 some of the pioneers conceived the idea that a trading point established in that vicinity would be a profitable investment and eventually merge into a thriving business center. The first post-office was established 1881. Chautauqua was one of the trading points and shipping stations for stock, on the Osage line. For months cattle are shipped from here by the train loads.

One of the main points of benefit of this town was the quality of water in the numerous springs, from which the town derives its name. They developed the springs, built a large hotel and bathhouse near the springs. They also bottled the spring water and sold it. The business included a livery barns, bath houses, general merchandise stores, lumber yards, restaurant, bakery, drug store, schools, hotels and bank The Chautauqua area also had an oil boom in the early 1900's. Chautauqua still has a post office and a store. The Chautauqua Springs have been renovated by the owners and a lovely park provided for picnics or just pleasurable outings.

CLOVERDALE was established in the early 1870 in Caneyville township on the road between Grenola and Cedar Vale. The town had a large general and notions, and has his store nicely arranged. In 1881, he was married to Miss N. E. Stevens, of Peru. They have one son -- Orie.

C. B. SIPPLE, M. D., was born in Delaware in 1851. In 1853, his parents emigrated to Michigan, locating at Niles, where he remained until 1864. Thence to Iowa, locating at Hamburg, Fremont County, and read medicine a part of the time until 1869, when he attended the medical department of the State University at Ann Arbor, Mich., until 1873. In the winter of 1874 - 75, he attended the St. Louis Medical College, and graduated in the spring of 1875. He then came to Kansas, and commenced the practice of medicine in Peru, and also engaged in the drug trade. Since his settlement here he returned to Iowa, thence to Michigan, and for a time was in Chicago, engaged in the practice of his profession. He then returned to Peru, where he again resumed the practice of medicine. In the winter of 1882, in company with I. Hillman, he put in a fine stock of drugs at Peru. They are having a large trade, and the Doctor is doing a large business in his practice. In the spring of 1883, he was appointed Postmaster. He was married in 1880, at Independence, Kan., to Miss Della Closson, of Chautauqua County. They have one daughter - Barbara. He is a member of Sedan Cornet Band, and is the examining physician of Chautauqua County for the Government.

J. D. STEVENS, M. D., was born in Harrison County, Ind., in 1836. In 1860, he emigrated to Vincennes, Knox Co., Ind., where he remained about five years, and commenced the study of medicine, finishing his course at the Miami Medical College, of Cincinnati, in 1867. He then located at Russellville, Lawrence Co., Ill., and began the practice of medicine. In 1874, he returned to Indiana, locating in Davis County. At the end of two years, he emigrated to Kansas, locating at Peru, where he has since been engaged in the practice of his profession, meeting with good success. He was married in 1856, to Miss M. A. Johnson, of Indiana. They were blessed with eight children, seven of whom are living -- Thomas A., Nancy E., Dora K., J. C., Abbie A., Mattie M., Edgar M., the seventh child, and Maggie A. In 1878, his wife died, and he married again in 1879 to Miss Mary D. Jackson, of Topeka, Kan. He is a member of Peru Lodge, No. 106, I.O.O.F.

F. THOMAE, merchant, was born in Saxen, Germany, in 1844. He was brought up there, learning the locksmith's trade, which he followed until 1866, when he emigrated to America, remaining about eight months in the State of Indiana. Thence went to Hancock County, Ohio, where he remained four years, and was employed as a salesman. In 1870, he emigrated to Kansas, locating in Howard County, and located a claim on Section 24, Township 34, Range 12. He was eighty-five miles from a railroad, and for six weeks during the first year had no mail, and then finally hired a man to take the mail through to the nearest post office. In the fall of 1871, he sold his place and put in the first stock of groceries and queensware in Peru, which business he has carried on since. He has added boots and shoes and built up a large trade, and is one of the best business men in the place, understanding the details of trade thoroughly. In December, 1882, he was married to Miss S. Sawyer, of Texas. He is a member of the Masonic order, and of Peru Lodge, No. 106, I.O.O.F.

CHAUTAUQUA SPRINGS.

This little city sprang into existence August 10, 1881. The presence of mineral springs, highly celebrated for the medical properties of the waters, was the chief incentive to its starting.

The place is situated in the south part of Chautauqua County, about eight miles south of the city of Sedan, and one mile from the picturesque Indian Territory. Its surroundings are beautiful, lying as it doses on the brink of a small rocky canon, a branch of Turkey Creek, from which stream it is a short distance. The landscape is interestingly diversified with hill, canon and rocky cliff, and is covered with a dense growth of shrub and timber. The city lies in the midst of a grove of forest trees, much of the timber being allowed to remain, giving it the appearance of a city in the woods.

The first house erected on the site belonged to B. F. Bennett, which he used for a drug store. Following this, during the fall, and in almost consecutive order, was the establishment of a dry goods house, by T. J. Johnston, a livery barn by F. M. Fairbanks, dry goods store by Thomas Bryant, a grocery and provision store by Bennett & Binns, and a drug store by George Edwards. In February, 1882, "Dick" Foster opened a stock of hardware, which he sold to W. Williams, in September of the same year. About the same time C. C. Purcell began the drug business. A grocery store belonging to James Randall was opened in October 1881, and about the same time Mrs. Bush started a millinery establishment. James Sipples opened a dry goods store in August, 1882. Besides these, there are also two livery barns, two blacksmith shops, two wagon shops, and a saw mill, belonging to James Allreid, who began the business in December, 1881.

The first hotel was built by a man named Castleberry, who ran it about six months, and after changing hands several times, it is still used as a hotel, of which there are now three in the city. Two of these, the Ginn and Meeks houses, are small affairs; but the other, the Eagle Hotel erected in June, 1882, by James Ferguson, is the finest public house in the county. It is a large two-story stone structure, seventy feet long and forty feet wide, containing twenty-five rooms, having accommodations for about sixty guests. The house is constructed with long verandas on two sides, and on either floor. It stands on the slope of the canon, a few steps from the springs, and overlooks the deeper canon of Turkey Creek, and the beautifully timbered hills, stretching far away in the smoky distance, into the Indian Territory.

The original town site comprised eighty acres, one-half of which belonged to Dr. G. W. Woolsey, and the other half to Dr. T. J. Dunn to which additions of forty acres each were made by J. C. Kiles, Binns and B. F. Bennett, making a total in the town site of 200 acres. The place was incorporated as a city of the third class in February, 1882, and Thomas Bryant was elected Mayor; S. Booth, Clerk; I. H. Wilson, Treasurer; B. E. Atkinson, Marshall, and M. O. Shoupp, N. M. Lee, F. A. Fairbanks, E. Moore and S. Cheny, Councilmen.

At the regular city election held in April 1882, E. P. Moore was chosen Mayor; S. Booth, Clerk; I. H. Wilson, Treasurer, and F. A. Fairbanks, M. O. Shoupp, N. M. Lee, S. Cheny and C. E. Moore, Councilmen.

The educational advantages of the city are in common with those of the country district within which it is included, the district having been organized and the house built in 1880. It is situated outside of the city limits, a short distance. Religious services are held at periodical times by the Baptist, Methodist, United Brethren and Church of Christ denominations in the schoolhouse, there being no regular church building provided.

The press has only a brief history at the place, only one attempt at journalism having been made. This was the establishment of the paper called the Chautauqua Springs *Spy*, on May 19, 1882, by C. E. Moore and L. G. B. McPheron, and is a seven-column folio, independent in politics, and has a circulation of 350 copies.

THE SPRINGS.

The main attraction in the city and the cause which gave rise to its building, is the presence of the mineral springs. These springs are highly valued on account of the medical properties contained in the waters, which are regarded invaluable in the cure of a variety of chronic sores and other diseases. The curative properties of these waters are known, not only through medical and chemical analysis, but are also attested by the apparently miraculous cures effected by their experimental use and application in many instances.

The discovery of these springs was made in 1873, by Dr. Minna, a physician who practiced in the vicinity at that time. It was his custom, when riding by, to drink of the water, and although recognizing the presence of mineral taste in them, yet made no further analysis. His belief during all this time, however, was that possibly, there were in these same waters medical ingredients that might prove valuable in the healing of diseases. In the latter years of his life the Doctor was afflicted with dropsy, and for a long time was under the treatment of medical skill, which he derived little benefit.

Finally the physicians gave up the case as incurable, and the old Doctor turning to the scriptural injunction of "Physician heal thyself," concluded, as a last hope, to try the waters which he had discovered. A quantity of the water was brought, of which he made frequent use and application, and from which he believed himself to experience much benefit. But the old man had too long been weighed down with the wasting disease, and the "treatment of physicians," to ever hope to regain health from any cause, and at length passed away, leaving, as a testimonial, his belief that had he begun the use of the water in time, he would have succeeded in removing the disease, and been restored to health.

Nothing was done toward making further test of these mineral springs until opened by Dr. G. W. Woolsey in August, 1880. The spring is neatly and substantially walled up, and is constructed with a large basin for holding the water, the whole being covered by a commodious spring house, tastefully built paved with flag rock, and conveniently seated with benches. An analysis of the waters was made by practical chemists of some note, of the cities of St. Joseph and Kansas City, showing the water to contain, in different proportions, iron, potassium, salts and magnetic gas.

While excavating the earth, in opening up the spring, the workmen struck upon rocks, standing upright, and arranged in a sort of basin shape, presenting evidence that it had been the handiwork of man, and giving rise to the theory that perhaps one day these waters were known to some Indian tribe, who made use of them in their primitive way, for the curing of disease.

The curative properties of these springs is as yet but little known, and it is safe to predict that when their efficacy shall become known to the world, and a thorough test is made, hundreds will flock in to partake of the benefits of the healing fountain.

The city as yet presents an appearance of newness, the most of the houses being unpainted and scattered.

The population of the town at this time numbers about 300, to which addition is being made by the incoming of settlers almost constantly.

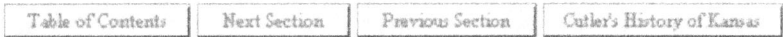

LOOKING BACK TO YESTERYEAR
SEDAN TIMES-STAR
August 12, 1954
Transcribed by Freida Wells

Chautauqua County History
Chautauqua First Baptist Church Struck By Lightning
by Louise McElroy

A bolt of lightening at three o'clock in the morning August 6, struck a double tragedy in the little town of Chautauqua, Kansas. The entire town and country side was awakened by and explosive report as the lightening struck 'somewhere.' Twenty minutes later there was question about the location. Black smoke was being belching from all openings in the First Baptist Church. In a few minutes the alarm was spread and practically the entire population came to help. It was hopeless. One of the first arrivals said, "The whole inside of the church looked like whirling rolls of fire.- We stayed back for fear of an explosion- when the roof fell in the explosive report could be heard all over town or farther.

The Sedan and Chautauqua Fire Department were soon at the scene of the fire but the blaze had gained so much headway in so short a time that all efforts were fertile. Not a single item was saved.

In the year 1904-05 Charlie Hampton built the native stone building. The first business to open within this structure was opened by J. M. Gwaltney. An old souvenir from the store reads, J. M. Gwaltney Hardware, Garage and Harness, Chautauqua, Kansas. Phone 48. In 1932 Mr. Gwaltney moved his store to Sedan. Between the years 32-39 a number of other business men occupied the store. George Fox had a garage for some time, followed by others in the garage business. Later, Frank Clark opened a been parlor and dance hall here. It was at the close of his venture that the most unusual history of the old landmark began.

A headline in the Historical Edition of the paper on September 25, 1941 read like this: Former Dance Hall Becomes Church. The story follows, telling of how thirteen charter members in 1939 led by their Pastor, Rev. Bob Maultsby, gave the beer parlor and dance hall a face-lifting which was so far reaching that only eternity can tell the results.

Five years later than the building date (1939) the story was different. There was now an enrollment of 74 in Sunday school and the building had been divided into an auditorium and six class rooms.

The chapter on record August 6, 1954, would read like this: There are now 77 members. The former member who have moved away and called for their letters would run this number far over the hundred mary. There are two ordained Ministers out in the filed who grew up in this church. Through gifts of love and sacrifice we have the following equipment: Twenty-seven Missouri pine pews with matching pulpit, eight nice stoves to warm the building, ceiling fan and smaller fans, two nice pianos, all types of literature and materials for the enjoyment and learning of the younger children. We have just bought new songbooks for the church. This is the only history now. The insurance taken out a number of years ago, would not cover anything like all the equipment.

The early morning of august 6, will be remembered by the church at the mooring of the Black Smoke Two hours after the lightening struck, the church was a smoldering heap of charred bricks and stones. The hopes and efforts of fifteen years gone up in smoke. The last of the observers some a part of the first thirteen members turned with tear filled eyes toward their homes.

Gloom didn't darken the sprits of this group for very long. As you talk with the various member you will hear such remarks as, "We've always been a group that made up in faith what we lacked in money or other things." "We'll not miss a service-we ill meet in the highschool building until we can do otherwise." The attitude of the entire church could be summed up in the words of some of the older members as they talked and said, "There is nothing so bad but what it could have been worse-just suppose that had been house with the father, mother and several small children asleep in different rooms."

Plan are already underway to rebuild the church. The faith of this group has spread to others who were not members. Some express their thoughts in this way, "We do not have so much money but we will be glad to donate labor as soon as you begin to rebuild." Money donations have started coming in from others. This faith like the mustard seed which could remove mountain, will soon bear fruits in the form of another building in Chautauqua, Kansas. The Rev. John Bowen, pastor, and his faithful members will probably be erecting a sign before too many months. The words will read something like "First Baptist Church." The vacant lit will not be vacant and there will be another chapter to write on the history of the old landmark.

CHAUTAUQUA

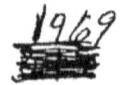
1969

Chautauqua lies in the three-mile strip
Between two old state borders;
Oklahoma, land of the Indian, and
Kansas of the longhorn herders.

Here were the coppery mineral springs,
Where the Indians gathered.
In 1880, tipped arrow wings,
Zoomed by, some of them feathered.

In the cemetery on the hill
The name Choteau is found.
Their ancestors built a trading post
On Oklahoma ground.

From Chautauqua's valley, across Jack Hill
And west to Tinker Hollow;
Beyond Devil's Canyon to the east
Are faint trails one may follow.

Moonshine Cave is not so far,
Nor the Map of Hidden Treasure.
I tell one of my little town
With a wealth of literary treasure.

Author— Louise McElroy

marshall, B. F. Atkinson; councilmen, O. F. Shoupp, N. M. Lee, F. A. Fairbanks, E. Moore, and S. Cheney.

CHAUTAUQUA SPRINGS

1961
(Research notes taken from the past)

As Chautauqua celebrates her birthday of 100 years, a description of the town would read as follows: One school which houses eight grades is now in use, the former high school. High school students go to Sedan or Peru. Three churches, Church of Christ, Assembly of God, and Baptist, serve the spiritual needs of the people. Parkers' Grocery and Service Station and Hills' Grocery and Service Station, Greer's Port of Entry and Service Station, Darnall Brothers Oil Well Serviceing, Padgett's Oil Drilling, a Post Office, and a City Hall where a mayor and the Councilmen meet regularly, make up the businesses. There is a population of 186 according to the 1960 census. Highway 99 skirts the western edge of the town thus enabling all citizens to find ready service of doctors, dentists, or other professional services in Sedan.

Locations of older buildings have become the sites of new homes, remodeled homes, and business buildings. The cemetery has been fenced and fronted by a silverdale stone nameplate and gateway. The cemetery has become an association and has been added to the tax rolls and given the number 13.

The residents of Chautauqua County readily avail themselves of the picnic facilities offered by the area sourrounding the Bulah Lake which is only a few miles southeast. Weekends find motorcades of cars bearing boats, swimmers, and tired workers, all lake bound for a bit of relaxation and fresh air. Former Chautauqua merchants, Ella and Stanley Friend, operate a lakeside grocery and supply store in the Hickory Hill addition on the Chautauqua side of the Hulah Lake. The Friends, Parkers, And Hills offer all variries of bait for the convenience of area fishermen.

Residents of Chautauqua and the area surrounding the mineral springs feel that the early Osage Indian who selected this site for his big summer "get-togethers", held in the out-of-doors, chose well. The natural beauty of the bluff lined valley, the cool air-conditioning afforded by the fresh spring waters and hugh transpiring sycamore, oak, and elm, all situated on a sandy soil, create an ideal location for a prolonged summer Chautauqua, be one Indian or otherwise. The Honorable Edward Janquins, a member of the 1875 Kansas Legislature, upon finding himself so confronted by a beautiful setting so much like that of his home area around Chautauqua Lake, New York, chose well when he named the little town of Chautauqua Springs, as well as the County of Chautauqua. Even today, an air of culture in music, art, writing, and preservation of early American furniture, glass, china, and relics of the past is strongly rooted in the area surrounding the springs. As a living monument to the Great Osage Trail, "Black Dog Trail", skirting the southern edge of Chautuauqa Springs and stopping in memory at the springs for overnight before going on towards the Leahy Crossing near Elgin, The Black Dog Trail Museum owned by the Parkers now stands with open doors to researchers.

Prentis, Noble   And
History of Kansas -
c. 1908: pages 323-324, 248 (map)

Baughman, Robert W.
Kansas Post Offices
Kans. State Historical Society
Topeka: c. 1961

Chautauqua County was organized in 1875 and the County seat was Sedan. This county was created out of a portion of what was first Godfrey County, named after Bill Godfrey, a noted trader among the Indians. Then it was later named Howard County in honor of Major-General O.O. Howard, for his efforts in behalf of the Union.

Chautauqua County, New York was the former home of Hon. Edward Janquins, a member of the Kansas Legislature in 1875 from Howard County, who introduced the bill which divided Howard into Chautauqua and Elk. (There had been a bitter county-seat war for an extended time.) Hence, from his native place the county derives its name.

However, it is interesting to note that the name originally given (in 1885) to Howard County was Godfrey and the name was changed to Seward in 1861. In 1867, the Legislature, ignoring the former names, created the county of Howard, which embraced all the territory of Seward and a five-mile strip additional on the weat.

Possibly adding to the growth of Chautauqua County was the following note: "Possibly the greatest discovery and development in Kansas in 1894 was in the oil and gas field. Oil and gas were discovered at Sedan, Thayer, Cherryvale, and other places. (This included Peru, Chautauqua, and other places in the County.)

*The post office of Chautauqua was organized on October 3, 1881 and George T. Edwards was the first appointee as post master. As of January 1, 1976, the office is still in active state and Mrs. Harold (Mary Rector) McDowell is post master.

Darla, I am adding a personal note: I remember that in 1944, a Mr. George Edwards was post master and served for years. Later, I remember his wife, Maggie Edwards serving in the office for many years. It seems that I read or heard that Maggie served the office for at least 15 years but I could be mistaken. I am sending along a plain, free-verse item I wrote concerning Maggie and her wonderful ways with the people. I never like to close a helpful item which I do for any person without adding the thought which you will find below.

"In 1853, Pamela Cunningham was Director of the Mount Vernon Ladies Association for the restoration and preservation of Mount Vernon, Washington's home."-----"Let one spot in this grand country of ours be safe from change. Upon you rests this duty."

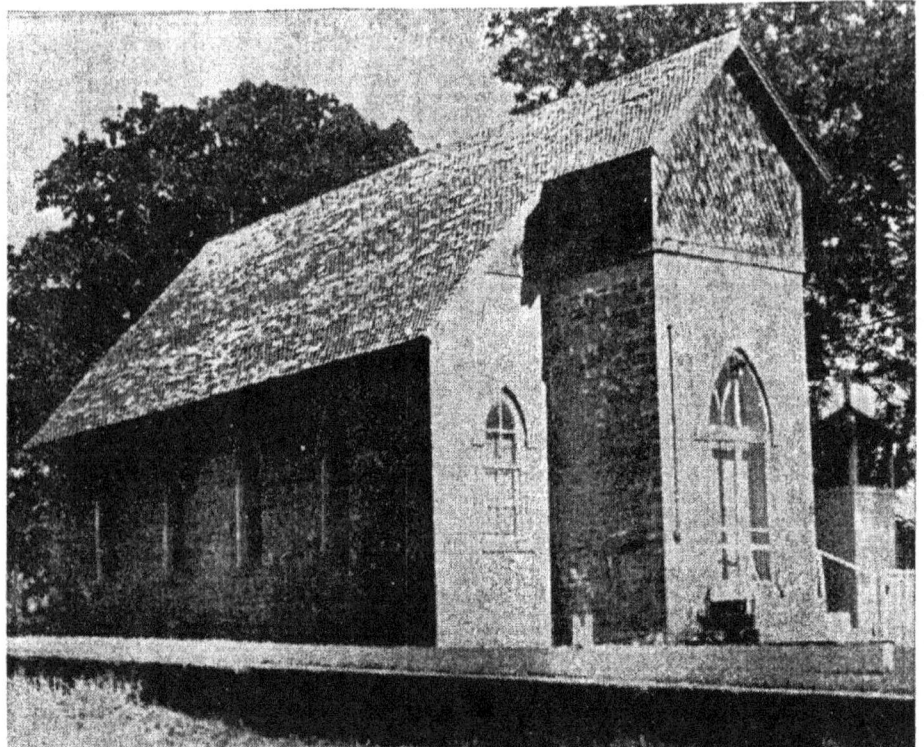

OCK CHURCH — This church building in Chautauqua is a picturesque example of the lasting qualities of stone masonry. Built around the turn of the century, services are still being held regularly at the church. Rev. B. E. Mowery is the pastor.

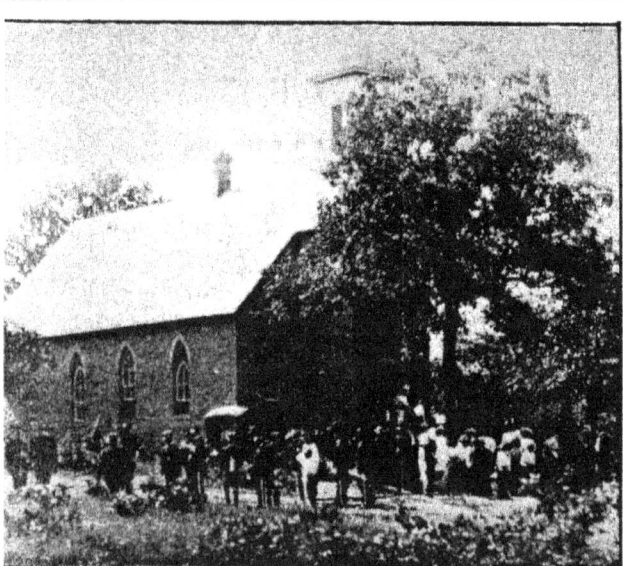

The Chapel of the Trails-Photo credit Louise McElroy

by Teresa Morrison

One of the most lasting landmarks today is the Chapel Of The Trails, located on Wilderness Trail-East Wing, two blocks east of Highway 99 in the south part of Chautauqua, Kansas. The chapel is always open and visitors are welcome to pray or meditate.

This sandstone church, built during the later part of 1886-87, was constructed of stone from the quarry northwest of town and located on the Joseph Slates farm, later know as the the Fred Burger farm.

Since the church was rather small, the dedication service was held at the Chautauqua Grade School, also new at that time. Reverend Eldridge delivered the sermon, assisted by the Methodist minister. Throughout the day, visitors viewed the new church grounds, spread picnic lunches and heard music furnished by local bandsmen.

Stop in at Steve's 99 and ask for directions to view this landmark.

wn

n attempted to
. They would
ines down in
old Robber's

ery quiet town
one can watch

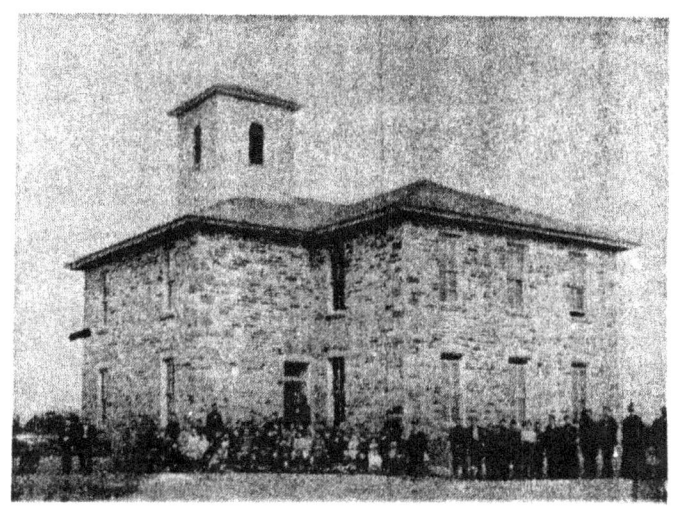

1892-Grade School built by Arthur Jay States.

CHAUTAUQUA

Chautauqua lies in the three-mile strip
Between two old state borders;
Oklahoma, land of the Indians, and
Kansas of the longhorn herders.

Here were the coppery mineral springs,
Where the Indians gathered.
In 1880, tipped arrow wings,
Zoomed by, some of them feathered.

In the cemetery on the hill
The name Choteau is found.
Their ancestors built a trading post
On Oklahoma ground.

From Chautauqua's valley, across Jack Hill
And west to Tinker Hollow;
Beyond Devil's Canyon to the east
Are faint trails one may follow.

Moonshine Cave is not so far,
Nor the Map of Hidden Treasure.
I tell one of my little town
With a wealth of literary treasure.
   --Louise McElroy

Krazy Kent's Star Restaurant
"Sedan's Largest Restaurant"
319 W. Main, Sedan, Ks.   725-5244
Open Daily 10:30 am - 9:00 pm

FTD   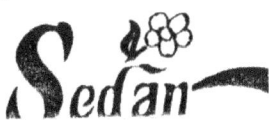   AFS

Sedan

CHAUTAUQUA RURAL HIGH SCHOOL FIRST IN STATE IN B CLASS SCHOOLS

(Research done by Journalism Director Louise McElroy, Sedan High School. Taken from files of Sedan Times Star, 1927 and personal interviews with Mr. and Mrs. Harold McDowel Chautauqua, KS and Duane Burger, son of Fred Burger, one of the 1927 team.)

Chautauqua Rural High School basketball players are the winners in Class B in the state finals, victors from a field of 248 Class B schools in the state of Kansas. The team was accompanied to Topeka by Coach Longhofer and Superintendent Andrews. They played March 18 and 19, a Friday and Saturday, by meeting four strong teams, two of which had not been defeated and two with only one defeat each for the season.

The winning team was composed of the following; Captain Donald Remmy, Wesley Fuller, Clarence Lane, Joe Dunn, Jack Stabler, Birl Stevens, Ormand Hamilton, George jack, and Fred Burger.

Sidelights noted are that Fuller was injured in the first game and was unable to play in the second. Also, that in the second game, Captain Remmy tossed in 15 of the total 22 points for Chautauqua.

Statistics:
First game	24-17	over Esbon
Second game	22-21	over Perry
Third game	27-18	over Ellis
Fourth game	33-13	over Williamsburg (previously undefeated)

After returning to Chautauqua the town gave the boys a banquet attended by approximately 300 people. All the honors and trimmings which a small place could afford were extended to the team of hardworking farm and oilfield boys, students of Chautauqua Rural High, who had gone all the way to the state Capital and brought home a First to their little near state-line community.

NEW CREDIT ASSOCIATION FOR COUNTY

(Taken from The Sedan Times-Star, November 12, 1936)

The retail merchants of Chautauqua county took a step forward this week when they organized a Retail Credit Association for this trade territory. The need for such an organization has been felt for some time but no one seemed to be willing to take the initiative to start the machinery for perfecting such an organization. For several weeks a group of merchants working in cooperation with the Sedan Chamber of Commerce have been making a study of Credit Organization. Mrs. Grace French who has been employed in the Crawford County Retail Credit Association office has been in Sedan interviewing merchants and helping in preliminary organization plans.

Fourteen merchants of the county have signed cards to give the organization a trial for one year.

Monday night a group of these merchants met at the Baird Funeral home and perfected organization plans to launch the organization in this county. Roy L. Harmon was elected president of the new association and the following Board of Directors were named: A.S. Baird, Lowell Ecker, Frank Harmon, Horace Dungan, and Dr. E. A. Marrs. It is planned to name enough directors to complete the list as soon as representatives from other sections of the county can be interviewed.

Mrs. Grace French will worth with the board during the next few weeks to get the new association functioning. An office will be secured at once and she will begin the task of compiling 4000 credit ratings on persons in this territory. The association has already joined the state association and has received much aid. The plan is to also join the National Association and have a connection with all associations in the matter of credit.

The association plan to hold regular meetings and to issue a bulletin from time to time which will be of interest to its members. No credit information will be given out from the association except to its members and all matters of credit will be held in strict confidence. At no time will anyone, not even members have access to files but will receive credit information only on certain individuals and under no consideration will the list be given to anyone. Those outside the association who receive information will be expected to pay for each report granted.

BUSY DAYS NOW AT ELGIN

Cattle Shipping Season Began Last Sunday

2500 CARS GO OUT THIS YEAR

Elgin a Dry Town for First Time in Fourteen Years—Many New Buildings There Now.

(Taken from the Friday, July 7, 1905 Sedan Times-Star)

These are stirring times at Elgin. There are no less than three distinct features of entertainment for the people to talk about. The cattle shipping season is just opening, the oil boom is on and the joints are closed tight. With three such prolific subjects to discuss there are no dull times at Elgin although everything is moving along without as much as even a ripple on the surface to indicate any unusual conditions

The first year, 1982-83, the school was held in the Campbell's home, because of limited space and increased enrollment, the school rented Hills' grocery building the second year. Thirty children attended school that year. As the school year drew to a close and some families moved away while others indicated they would not be returning, it was evident the large building was not expedient. So the Campbells purchased a house on Chautauqua Street in Chautauqua and began remodeling.

As this is being written, the third year of school draws to a close, and fifteen children are learning and growing together in the comfortable surroundings of a small, friendly town. Chautauqua has welcomed the Christian school with open arms and the Campbells have learned to love Chautauqua.

by Bernyce Campbell

Chautauqua School
T165

A school district known as Chautauqua Springs was established prior to 1874, and a log school house constructed in 1879 housed

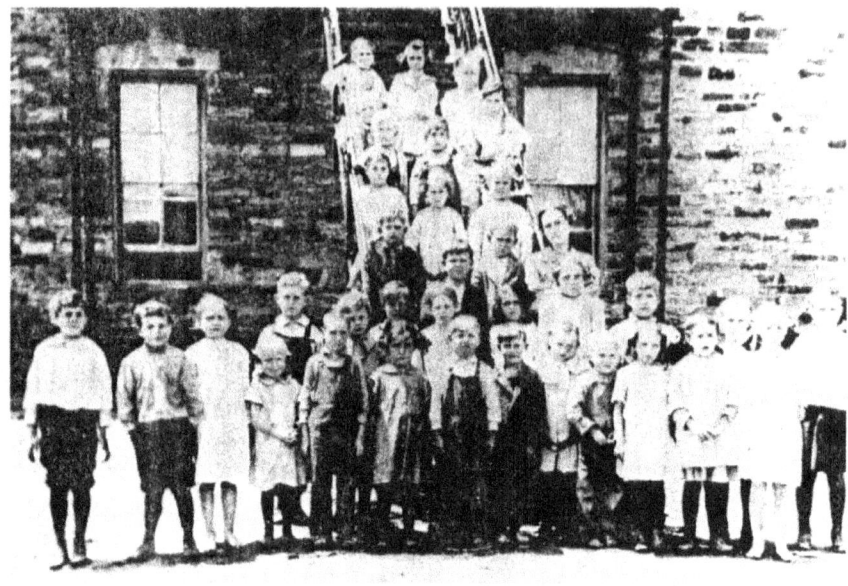

Chautauqua school in 1911. Second row, second from left, Myrtle (Tennent) Kelly; fourth from left, Mary (Tennent) Parker. Photo shared by Mary Parker.

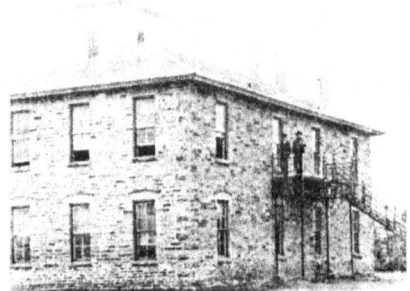

Old Rock School.

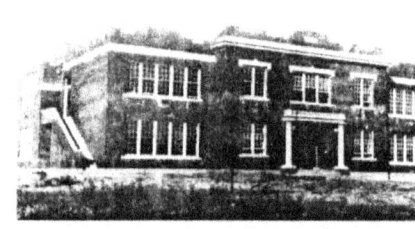

Chautauqua High School. Photo shared by Seba Childress.

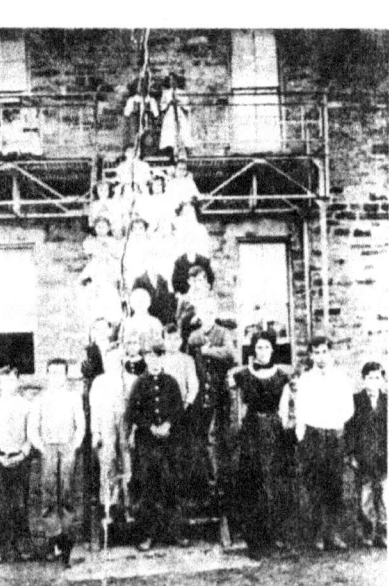

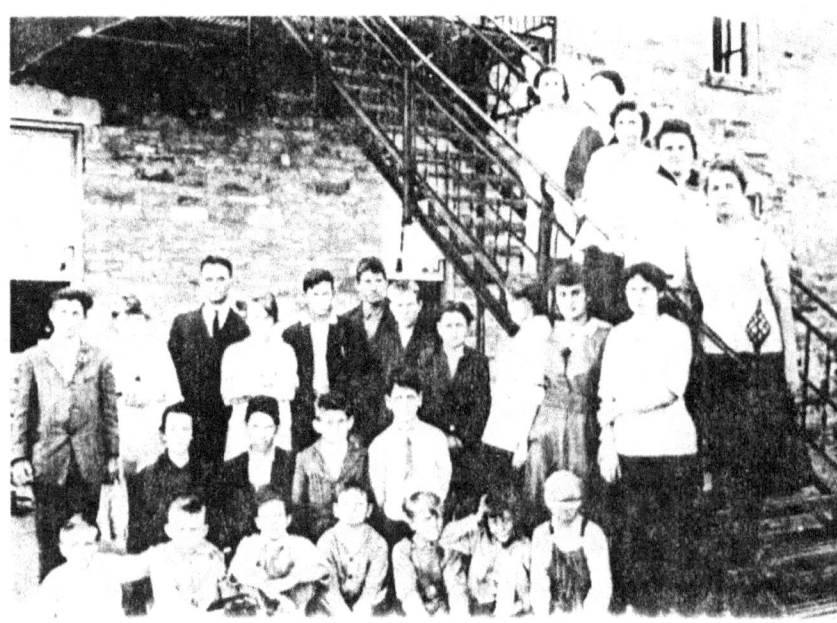

Chautauqua School in 1911-12. Bottom row, Frankie Burger, Mal Revard, Lucy Stabler (teacher), unknown, William Tyler, unknown; second row, Ralph Slates, Willard Runyon, third, Brice Sipple, Mart Edwards, Fred Wright, unknown, Merle Wade, Berlin Sipple; girls L-R, Ida Anderson, Alta Clingan, unknown, Marie Golden, Nina Clingan, unknown, unknown, Minnie L. Boulanger, Madeline Scott, Celeste Boulanger, Elsie Mitchell. Identification was made in 1974 by Minnie (Boulanger) Krepps and the picture was submitted by Louise McElroy. Other early day teachers were Hadely Fairley in 1912-13, and Bessie Pulliam in 1913-14.

69 pupils. School was maintained for three months that year at a total cost of $177.45. To raise the budget, one mill was levied against the taxpayers of the district

About 1880 – 1883 A.J. Slates, mason, and helpers began work on

The soil is the sandy loam, very rich and productive. The diversity of crops that may be raised in this locality is simply wonderful. Corn, wheat, cotton, barley, and in fact anything that can be raised any place in the United States can be raised here.

The rapidity with which the oil development has been carried in this field passes all belief.

On August 1, 1903, the first well in this field, Clark No. 1, was brought in. Excitement jumped to a fever heat. A man of some means was the only person that could afford to take a lease, thereby keepig out companies capitalized on hot air and operated by wind jammers. Today there are hundreds of wells within a radius of a few miles with an aggregate production of over 5,000 barrels per day. A person, by going to the top of a hill one mile north of town can, any day, see over 100 wells in operation. And while there is lots of land leased and being developed, there is a great deal yet that is fairly well proven.

The gas proposition is a settled question here also. Chautauqua is heated and lighted by gas, and there are a large number of gas wells that are capped and waiting for some enterprising manufacturer who wants cheap fuel to come in and take it. The Atchison Topeka and Santa Fe system runs in here and affords ample shipping facilities. If you have the inclination, energy, brains and money here is your opportunity for investment. Come and do it now.

Merchants of Chautauqua in 1905 were listed as follows: G. T. Edwards, dealer in general merchandise; Burgner-Bowman Lumber Co. W. C. Hulett, manager; The Chautauqua Bottling Works, D. B. Easly, manager; Meeker bros., dealers in general merchandise; J. A. Andrews at the Palace drug store; Hotel Byers, C. C. Byers Proprietor; Sipple and Hessert, butcher shop; Pete's short order restaurant.

Other Chautauqua firms in 1905 were: J. W. Harshbarger, attorney-at-law; Chautauqua Gas company, H. S. Gaines, manager; Chautauqua Bakery, S. C. Sproul, proprietor; Bowen and Leisure, butchers; the Citizens State bank; Strong and Fox, livery feed and sales stable; W. V. Cottingham, liveryman; Long-Bell Lumber company, W. W. Withers, manager; Southern Kansas Supply company, J. N. Carr, manager, R. W. Black, president; General merchandise, E. B. Glover.

Grade School Building at Chautauqua

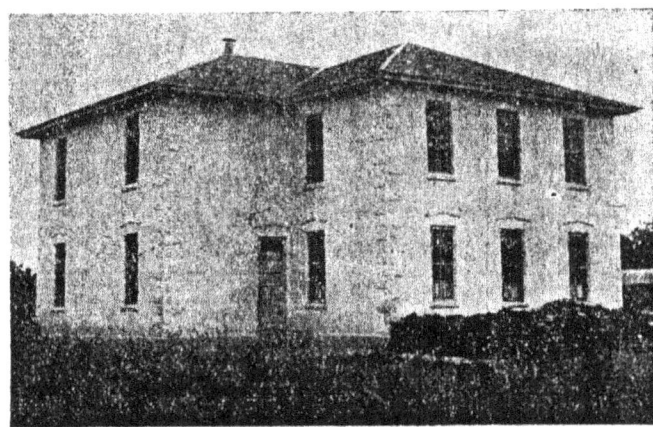

Photos by James Hadley

Above is the grade school building at Chautauqua. Teachers for the year 1940-41 were: Frances Coysh and Mercedes Holland.

Rural High School at Chautauqua

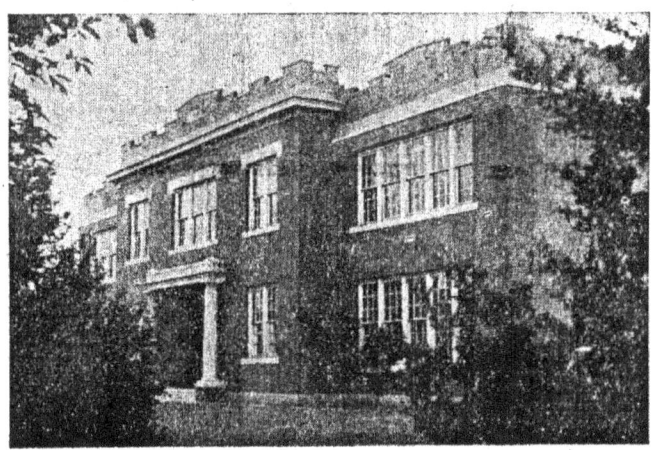

Photos by James Hadley

The fine building shown above houses the rural high school, located at Chautauqua. Teachers for the 1940-41 years were: J. H. Ulm, superintendent; Evelyn Ward and Floyd Hanson.

HOTEL BYERS

C. C. Byers, Prop.

Chautauqua can boast of just as good a hostelry as any in Southeastern Kansas. Large, spacious rooms, table the best market affords.

Mr. Byers has had years of experience in hotel keeping and no person could not truthfully say that he was not a decided success in that line. Mr. Byers has been in this community for a long time and has a host of friends. He was mayor of the city during the past two years.

The Byers has made itself solid with the commercial men and the oil men, as can be seen there every day. Traveling men come quite a distance every Sunday to take their weekly vacation at Chautauqua Springs and stop at the Byers.

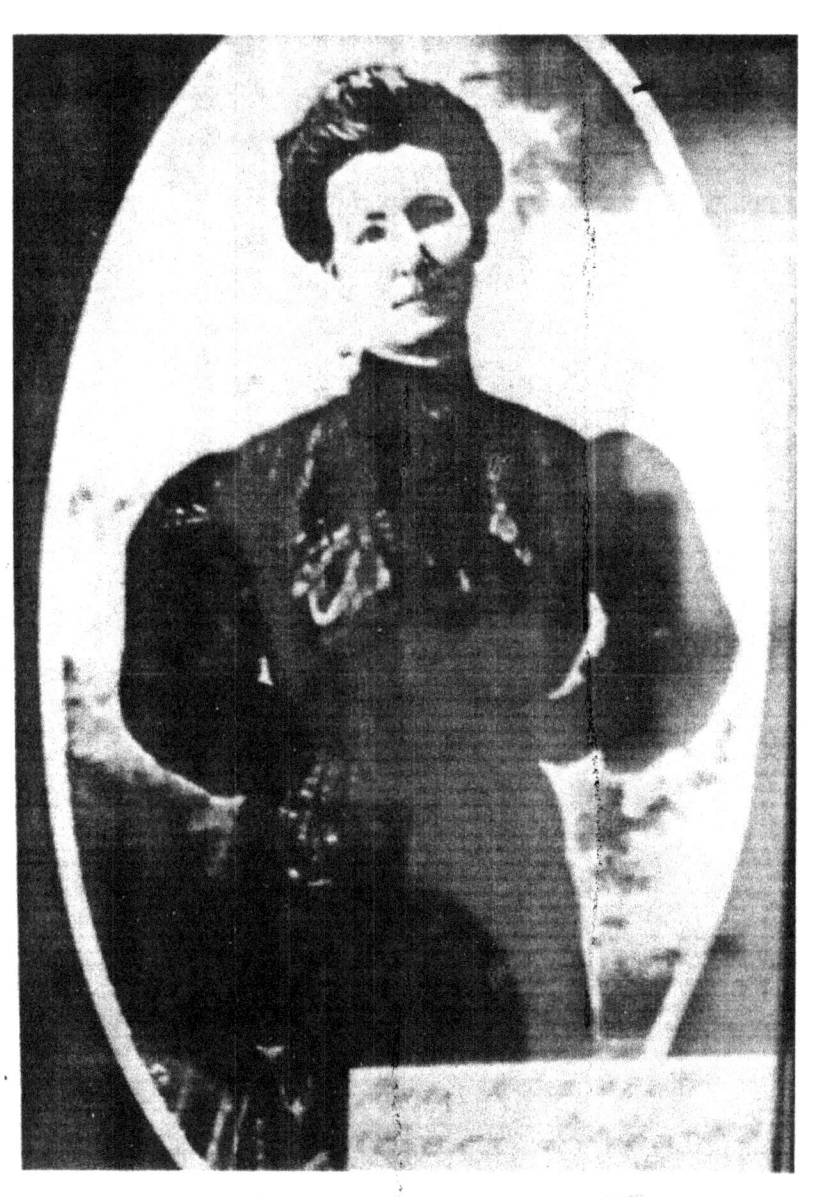

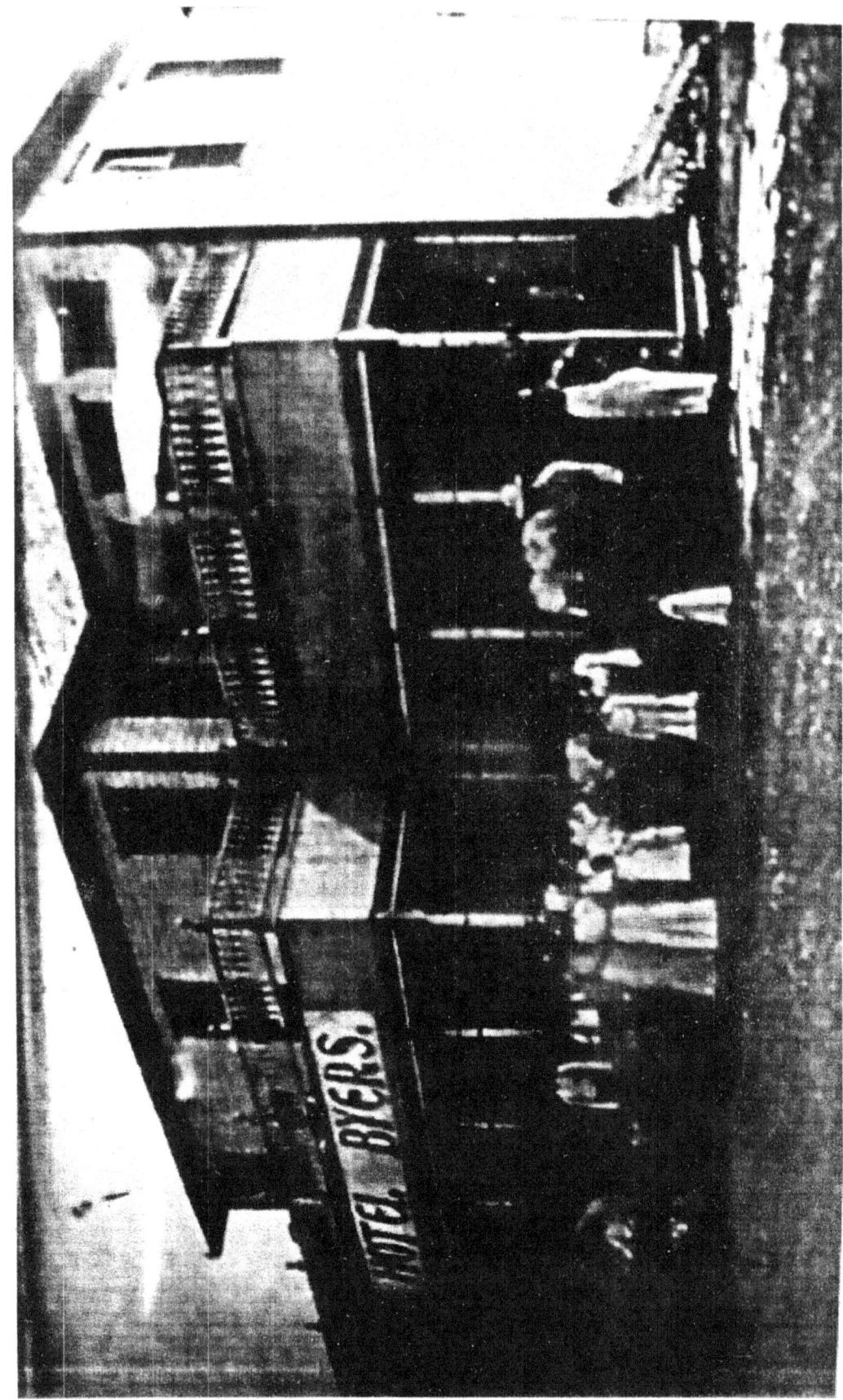

Lorna Doon, Chautauqua Pkwy

POST CARD

CORRESPONDENCE

NAME AND ADDRESS

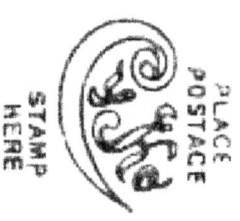

The Chautauqua Bath House
and
Bottling Works

Open at All Hours

The temperature of this water is 58 degrees Fhr., and the flow is 180 gallons per hour. The medicinal properties of this water is unsurpassed for bathing purposes and we are equipped to serve every one.

The management is arranging to construct a salt water lake, the water to be gotten from a "duster" that was recently drilled in.

The park in which this wonderful spring is situated is one of nature's most beautiful pieces of handiwork, embellished by all of the arts and devices of which the most resourceful men could give it.

The bottling works of itself is an institution that would do credit to a city many times the size of Chautauqua, and coupled with a supply of water that is as pure as the molten snow and has all the healing power of a modern apothecary shop, the combination is certainly one to consider.

When wanting the only liquid given by the all wise Creator, in any form whatever, call on us.

D. B. EASLY, Manager

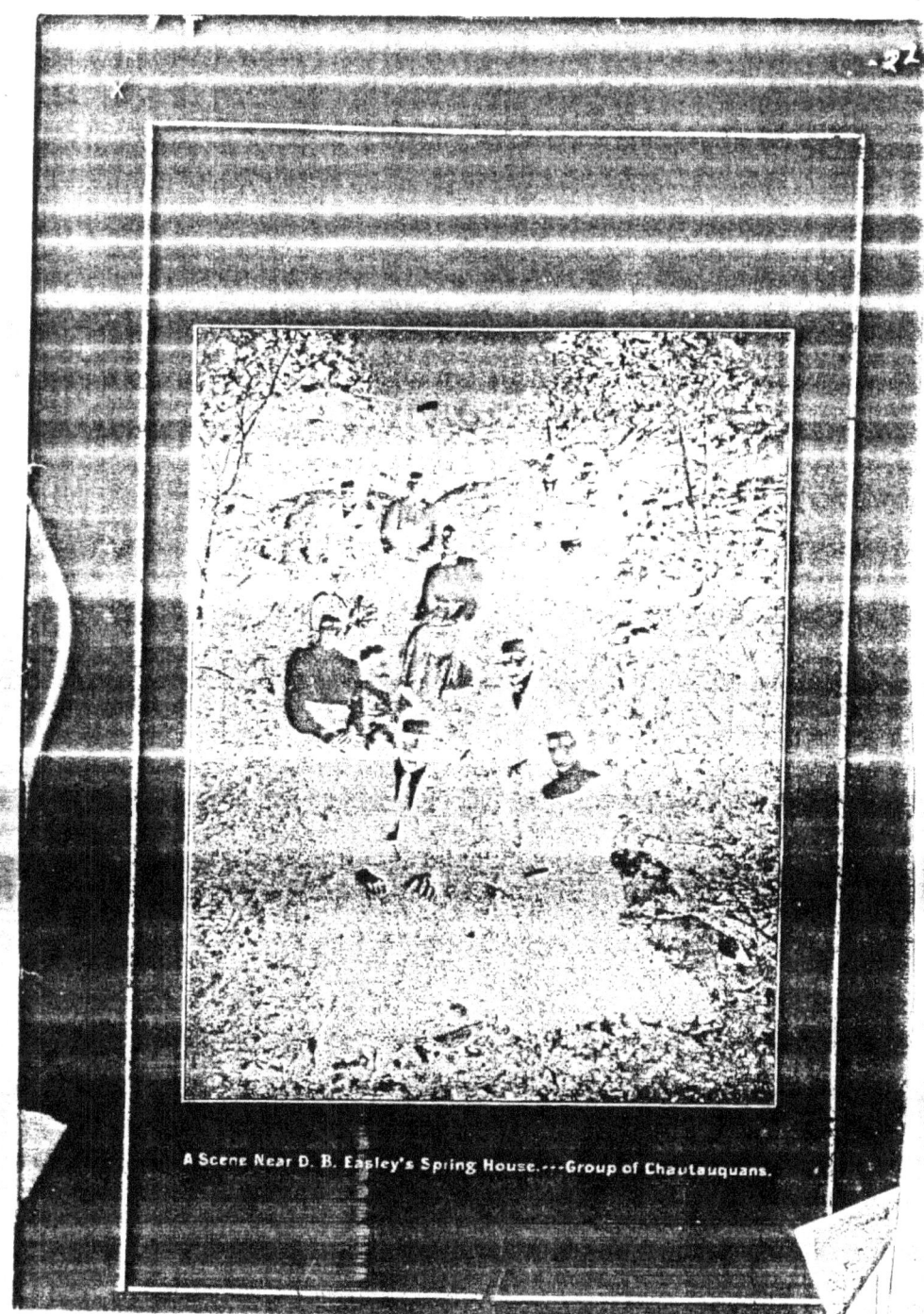

A Scene Near D. B. Easley's Spring House.----Group of Chautauquans.

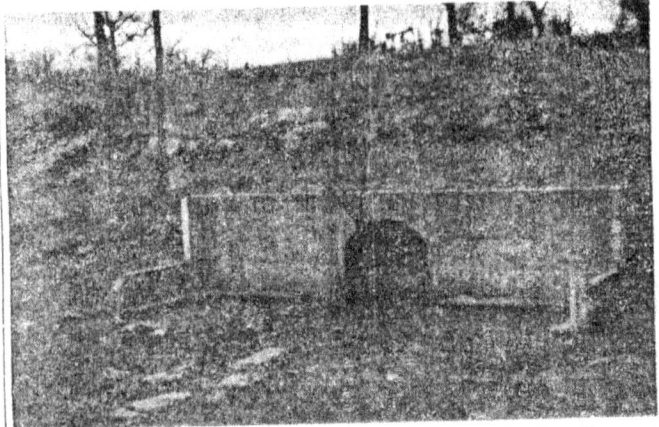

WELLS OF LIFE-EVER-FLOWING SOURCES
by Curt Parker

Many farmers and ranchers in parts of Chautauqua county, especially during droughts and periods of prolonged dryness, are very much in debt, not to banks or loan companies particularly, but to the natural springs. These springs, in many cases, water the farmer's family as well as his livestock. No matter how long it has been between rains, these "wells of life" have almost never been known to go dry, therefore they have been relied upon as an ever-lasting source of water.

Because these springs were not made by man, they have been here for hundreds of years. Some of them have articles around them which are very old. Sometimes it is possible to find relics of people who have been there to drink long ago. One might go hunting around a spring and find an arrowhead or some other artifact that was left there before the coming of the white man by Indians who chose a watered place for their temporary camp as they followed the various kinds of wild game across the plains. It is also possible that one might find a rusted bucket which was discarded by an early settler of the county. A spring was often the life-line of the pioneer.

At a natural spring, one can also find articles left there by people of modern times. Such things as shotgun shells or even money are found there because people become thirsty doing things like hiking or hunting for cattle.

Speaking of cattle—they use the springs for their water supplies too, as did long ago their ancestors, the buffalo. At many of such springs one might come upon anything in the form of animal wild-life drinking from the waters —if he is quiet upon his approach.

There are hundreds of such springs in southeastern Chautauqua county and very few of them have names or have been heard of by great numbers of people. These springs, especially those near the Oklahoma line, have a high mineral content.

One of these, the Chautauqua Springs, located in the city of Chautauqua, was once very famous. Mineral baths were featured at the Springs and the mineral water was shipped to all parts of the country.

Just follow any creek or gully long enough and it is more than likely that you will find one of these wells of life.

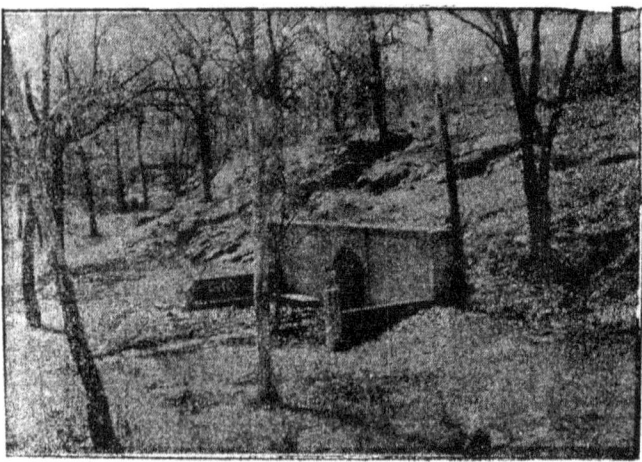

The Spring in Chautauqua—Photo credit Louise McElroy

Springs Were Big Asset to Chautauqua in Earlier Day

(Note: The following history of Chautauqua is reproduced from a booklet advertising the town published in 1905.)

Chautauqua Springs is a thriving little village of 600 inhabitants situated in the southern part of Chautauqua county, being only one and one half miles from the line dividing Kansas and the Osage reservation.

In 1881 some of the pioneers conceived the idea that a trading point, established at some place in that vicinity, which at even that early date was famed for its fertile valleys and rich pasture lands, would be a profitable investment, and eventually emerge into a thriving business center.

Their hopes have been realized and today Chautauqua is one of the best trading points and shipping stations for stock of all kinds, on the Osage line.

For years, during the shipping season, cattlemen from the immense pastures of the Osage reservation, found it advantageous to drive the stock to Chautauqua and ship. For months cattle are shipped from here by the train loads.

One of the main points of benefit of this town is the quality of water to be found in the numberless springs, from which the town derives its name. Ever since the Osage Indians were removed from Kansas to the present reservation, the healing power of this water has been known all over the central part of the United States.

Great bands of Indians, in the early days, bringing some noted chief or warrior to these springs to be healed were very common occurences. The springs have been cleaned out, renovated, furnished so that today, despite the great influx of people owing to the great oil fields being developed, it is the best advertisement through the central states that the city has.

Following is the chemical analysis of the Chautauqua Springs mineral water made by the state chemist in 1883: Calcium sulphate 4,047; calcium bicarbonate 3,849; magnesium 2,986; sodium 1,015; iron 1,455; sodium chloride 3,295; potassium sulphate 1,181; silica 1,633; magnesia bicarbonate trace; organic, violatile material 163 All quantities are in grains per gallon.

Chautauqua Springs

Chautauqua Springs is a thriving little village of 600 inhabitants situated in the southern part of Chautauqua county, being only one and one half miles from the line dividing Kansas and the Osage reservation.

In 1881 some of the pioneers conceived the idea that a trading point established at some place in that vicinity, which at even that early date was famed for its fertile valleys and rich pasture lands, would be a profitable investment, and eventually merge into a thriving business center.

Their hopes have been realized and today Chautauqua is one of the best trading points and shipping stations for stock of all kinds, on the Osage line.

For years, during the shipping season, cattlemen from the immense pastures of the Osage reservation, found it advantageous to drive the stock to Chautauqua and ship. For months cattle are shipped from here by the train loads.

One of the main points of benefit of this town is the quality of water to be found in the numberless springs, from which the town derives its name. Ever since the Osage Indians were removed from Kansas to the present reservation, the healing power of this water has been known all over the central part of the United States. Great bands of Indians, in the early days, bringing some noted chief or warrior to these springs to be healed were very common occurences. The springs been cleaned out, renovated, furnished so that today, despite the great influx of people owing to the great oil field being developed, it is the best advertisement through the central states that the city has.

The soil is the sandy loam, very rich and productive. The diversity of crops that may be raised in this locality is simply wonderful. Corn, wheat, cotton, barley, and in fact anything that can be raised any place in the United States can be raised here.

The rapidity with which the oil development has been carried in this field passes all belief.

On August 1, 1903, the first well in this field, Clark No. 1, which

Long-Bell Lumber Company

W. W. Withers, Manager

This company is one of the pioneer lumber concerns of the county. They have had yards in here ever since the county was first organized and their popularity is best evidenced by the amount of business they are doing.

In this yard one can find everything from a grain of sand to a walking beam.

All kinds of building material and rig timbers can be had here at terms that will favorably compare with the prices of any other yard.

Sipple & Hessert

When you want anything in the line of

Fresh, Salt or Cured Meats

We have an

Up-To-Date Shop

And handle everything usually found in a city market. Don't forget, here you get good goods

At Reasonable Prices

Opposite the Byers Hotel

Southern Kansas Supply Company

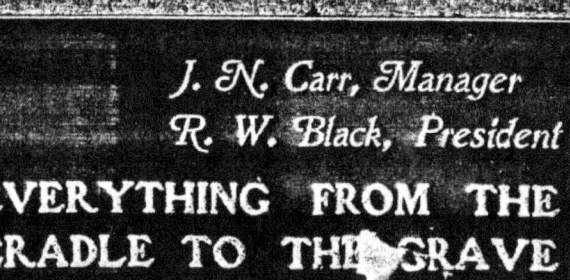

J. N. Carr, Manager
R. W. Black, President

EVERYTHING FROM THE CRADLE TO THE GRAVE

General Merchandise

W. O. Cottingham

LIVERYMAN

HERE is where the good teams and buggies come from.

HERE is where your horse, when brought in to be fed, will not go away hungry.

HERE is where, when you go away after paying your livery bill, you will not be mad.

HERE is a man who will give all that your horse is worth, if you want to sell.

Or in other words

We Treat You Right

Strong & Fox

New Livery Feed and Sales Stable

All kinds of live stock bought, sold or exchanged. Largest and most complete stock of high class vehicles, consisting of buckbnards, surreys, open and top driving wagons, also best rubber tired goods in the county.

Complete line of harnesses---single, light driving, farm and heavy team harness. Fly nets, dusters, halters, sweat pads, lap robes and whips.

We trade for, buy or sell anything in our line.

Chautauqua Bakery

S. C. Sproul, Prop.

We have the only

First Class Bakery

in the city, and bake and handle a Complete Line.

The confection department is an attractive feature. The above cut portrays the interior.

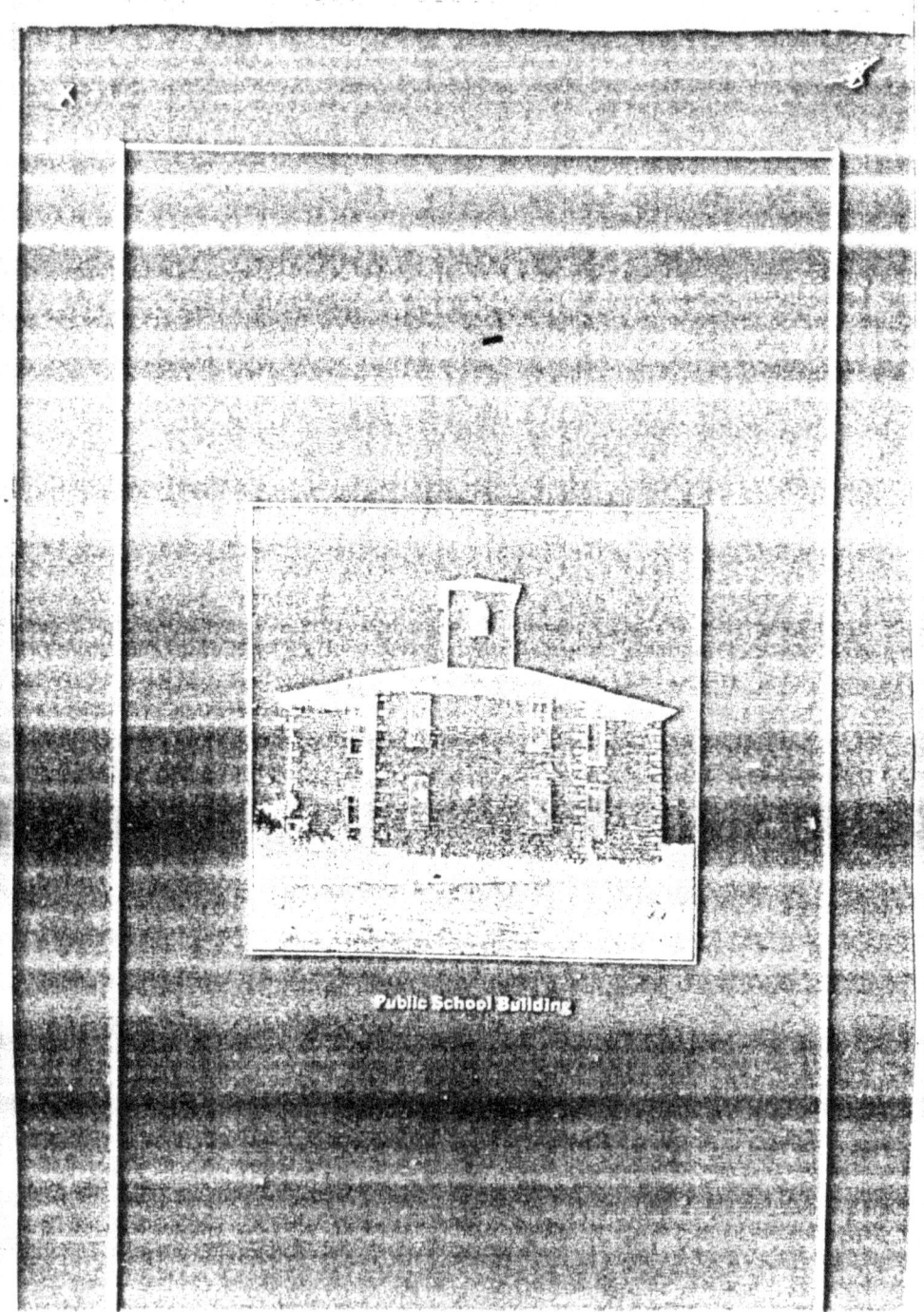

Public School Building

Bowen & Leisure

BUTCHERS

Leaders in

Oysters, Fish and Game in Season

We also buy

Good Beeves, Fat Hogs, Calves,

Chickens, Butter and

Eggs

We stand for FAIR AND COURTEOUS
TREATMENT, GOOD MEASURES
AND CORRECT WEIGHTS

Bread is the staff of life
but meat is the food from
which the staff is made

PETE'S SHORT ORDER RESTAURANT

When coming to our town
Don't forget to call at this place for

Good Meals and Quick Service

Open at All Hours

J. W. Harshbarger

Attorney-at-Law

Practice in all courts in Kansas

Real Estate and Insurance

Lease Work a Specialty

All kinds of Notarial work done

Chautauqua Gas Company

H. S. GAINES, Manager

We Have

Gas to Burn
Gas For Lights
Gas For Stoves
Gas For Drilling Purposes

We have enough gas to supply fuel for 25 factories.

Manufactors looking for cheap fuel would do well to write to us before locating.

Burgner-Bowman Lumber Co.

W. O. Hulett, Manager

Dealers in

Everything in Lumber
and Building Material

Brick

Lime

Sand

Cement

Paints and Oils

RIG TIMBERS A SPECIALTY

is reproduced on this page was brought in. Excitement jumped to a fever heat. A man of some means was the only person that could afford to take a lease, thereby keeping out companies capitalized on hot air and operated by wind jammers. Today there are hundreds of wells within a radius of a few miles with an aggregate production of over 5,000 barrels per day. A person, by going to the top of a hill one mile north of town can, any day, see over 100 wells in operation. And while there is lots of land leased and being developed, there is a great deal yet that is fairly well proven and can be had at a very nominal price by the right person, if they can show that they mean business and are not one of the many wild cat concerns.

The gas proposition is a settled question here also. Chautauqua is heated and lighted by gas, and there are a large number of gas wells that are capped and waiting for some enterprising manufacturer who wants cheap fuel to come in and take it. The Atchison Topeka and Santa Fe system runs in here and affords ample shipping facilities. If you have the inclination, energy, brains and money here is your opportunity for investment. Come and do it now.

For further particulars see, or write, C. R. WALTERHOUSE, Chautauqua, Kansas.

G. T. EDWARDS

Dealer in

GENERAL MERCHANDISE

The subject of this sketch was one of the first to see the advantages and prospects of Chautauqua Springs. Being a man of action, enterprise and push, he immediately embarked in the mercantile business, which he has successfully continued. Everybody who comes to Chautauqua knows that the name of Geo. T. Edwards is synonomous with fair, straightforward and upright dealing. Being one of the old settlers and of such sterling quality he has built up his trade to such extensive proportions that he has been compelled to add two 50-foot front buildings to keep pace with the fast increasing business and progress of the town and community.

Mr. Edwards, with the able assistance of his accomplished wife, has, for the past year, had charge of the Edwards Hotel. It has been remodeled and refitted until it is one of the best hotels on the Santa Fe system.

In the store Mr. Edwards is associated with his son, Mort, who can be found behind the counter at all times, during business hours, waiting upon the trade.

GENERAL MERCHANDISE
B. B. GLOVER

Dry Goods
Groceries
Hardware
Perfumes
Rugs and
Gloves
A Specialty of Shoes and Clothing

Meeker Bros.

Dealers in

General Merchandise

We Make a Speciality of

Oil Men's Furnishings

We cater to all of the country trade and heartily invite you to our store when you want to buy goods or sell produce.

We pay the HIGHEST market price in cash for all country produce.

Call On

J. A. ANDREWS

At the

Palace Drug Store

For

Drugs, Notions, Cigars,

Ice Cream Sodas,

In fact EVERYTHING that is usually found in a first class drug store.

Located in Jack's Block,
Chautauqua, Kas.

Hickory Hill, Okla.

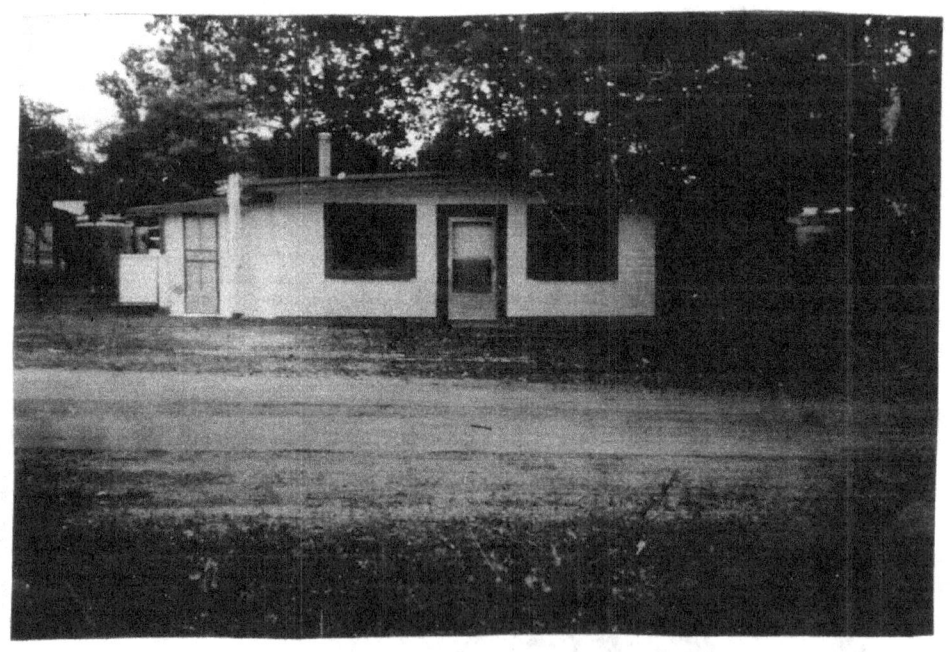

Before Page 48

Hickory Hill, OK.

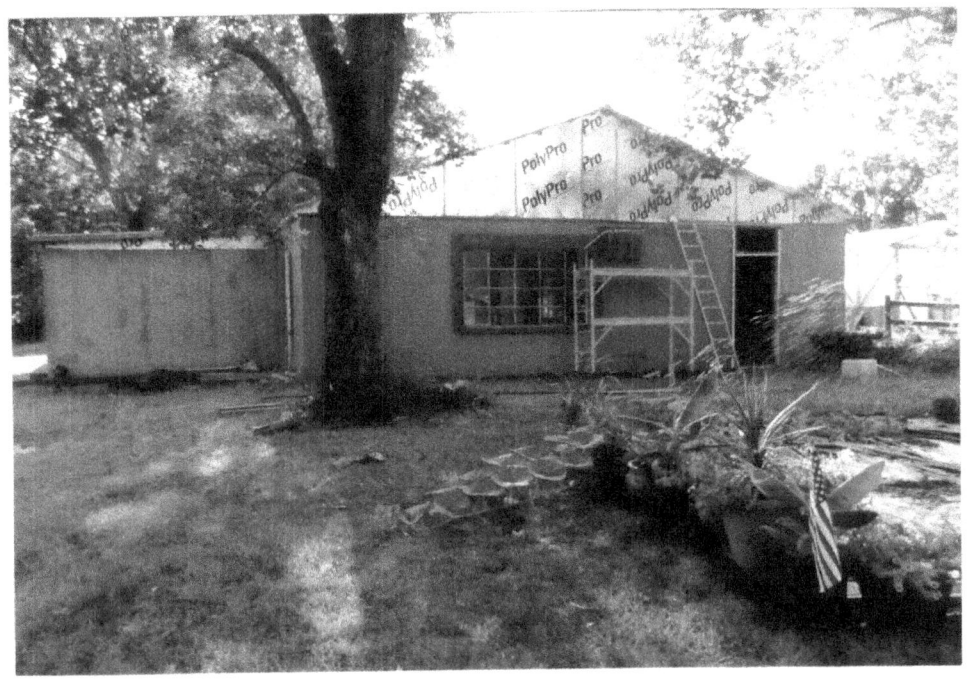

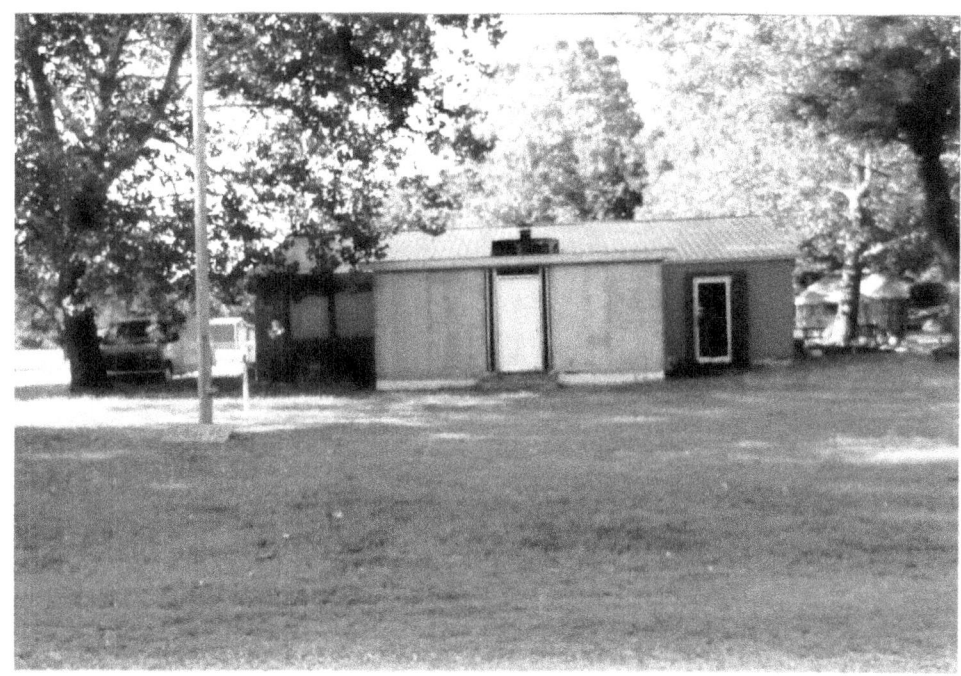

Hickory Hill Okla

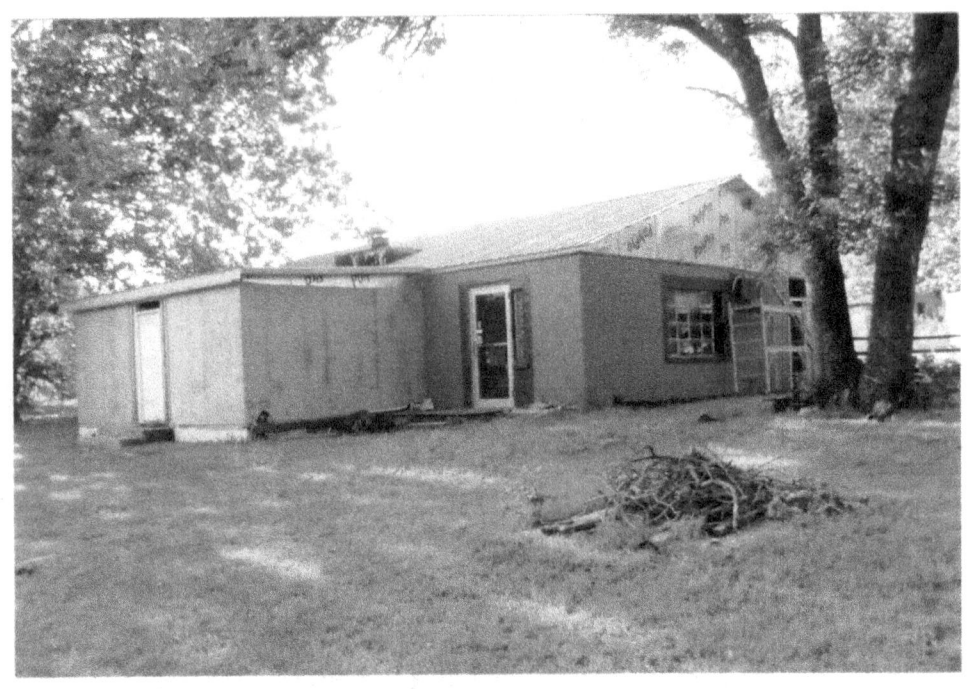

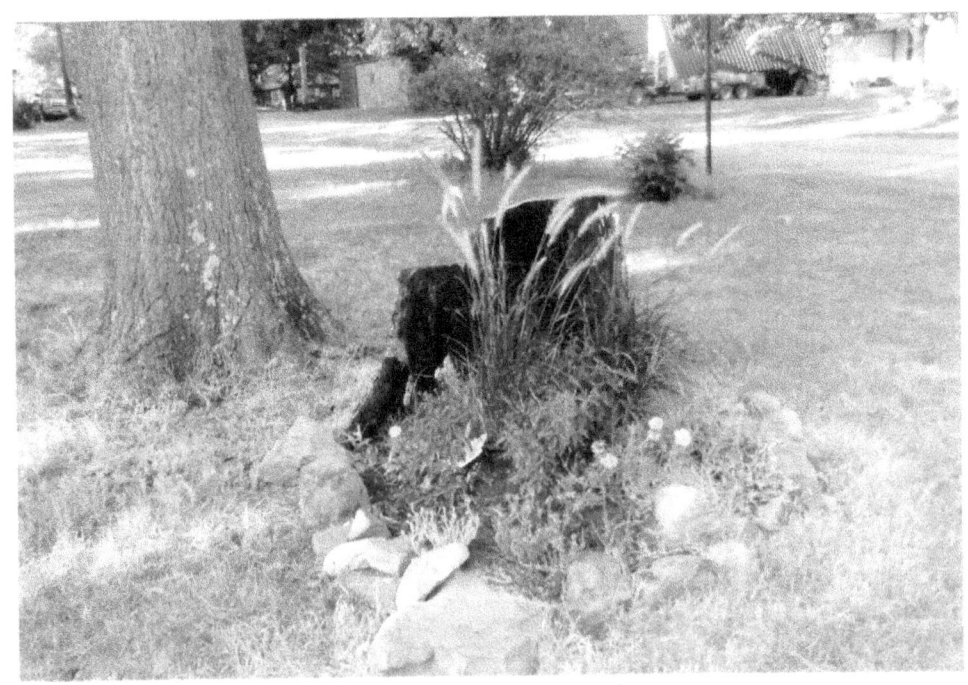